FAST FACTS FOR EVIDENCE-BASED PRACTICE

Implementing EBP in a Nutshell

About the Author

Maryann Godshall, MSN, PhD(c), RN, CPN, CCRN, CNE, is Assistant Professor at DeSales University in Center Valley, PA, and a CCRN in Pediatric Intensive Care (PICU) at Lehigh Valley Hospital Center, Allentown, PA. At DeSales University, Ms. Godshall teaches Pediatrics, Nursing Research, Health and Physical Assessment, Nursing Concepts, Evidence-Based Practice, and Senior Seminar. In addition, her responsibilities include syllabus development, course structure, and administration of all grades in-hospital clinical instructions, organization of laboratory and hospital orientations for students, orientation of pediatric adjunct faculty, plus the development, implementation, and facilitation of pediatric simulation experience. She has previously taught at Cedar Crest College (Allentown, PA), Northampton Community College and Lehigh County Community College. In addition to Ms Godshall's clinical PICU experience at Lehigh Valley Hospital, she has worked in Pediatrics, Pediatric Home Care, Neonatal Intensive Care (NICU), and Medical Surgical Telemetry in a variety of hospital settings. She is the coeditor with Dr. Ruth Wittman-Price of the *Certified Nurse Educator (CNE) Review Manual (2009-Springer,* in which she also authored a chapter. She has also written two chapters, "Caring for the Child with Cancer" and "Caring for the Child with a Chronic Condition or the Dying Child" and coauthored "Caring for a Child with an Integumentary Condition" in *Maternal-Child Nursing Care: Optimizing Outcomes for Mothers, Children, and Families,* coedited by Susan L. Ward and Shelton M. Hisley. She has written a chapter on pediatric disaster preparedness, entitled "Special Populations in Disasters: The Child and Pregnant Woman," in *Disaster Nursing: A Handbook for Practice,* coedited by Deborah S. Adelman and Timothy J. Legg. She has published eight journal articles and has given three national poster presentations about both pediatric and nursing education topics.

FAST FACTS FOR EVIDENCE-BASED PRACTICE

Implementing EBP in a Nutshell

Maryann Godshall, MSN, PhD(c), RN, CPN, CCRN, CNE

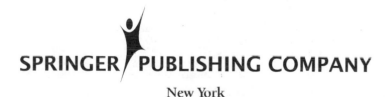

SPRINGER PUBLISHING COMPANY

New York

Springer Publishing Company, LLC
11 West 42nd Street
New York, NY 10036
www.springerpub.com

Acquisitions Editor: Margaret Zuccarini
Production Manager: Barbara A. Chernow
Cover design: David Levy
Composition: Agnews, Inc.

Ebook ISBN: 978-0-8261-0000-0

10 11 12 13/ 5 4 3 2 1

The author and the publisher of this Work have made every effort to use sources believed to be reliable to provide information that is accurate and compatible with the standards generally accepted at the time of publication. Because medical science is continually advancing, our knowledge base continues to expand. Therefore, as new information becomes available, changes in procedures become necessary. We recommend that the reader always consult current research and specific institutional policies before performing any clinical procedure. The author and publisher shall not be liable for any special, consequential, or exemplary damages resulting, in whole or in part, from the readers' use of, or reliance on, the information contained in this book. The publisher has no responsibility for the persistence or accuracy of URLs for external or third-party Internet Web sites referred to in this publication and does not guarantee that any content on such Web sites is, or will remain, accurate or appropriate.

Library of Congress Cataloging-in-Publication Data

Godshall, Maryann.
    Fast facts for evidence-based practice : implementing EBP in a nutshell / Maryann Godshall.
        p. ; cm.
    Includes bibliographical references and index.
    ISBN 978-0-8261-0567-7 (alk. paper)
    1. Evidence-based nursing.   2. Nursing—Research—Methodology.   I. Title.
    [DNLM: 1. Evidence-Based Practice—methods. WB 102.5 G589f 2010]
    RT81.5.G63   2010
    610.73—dc22
                                                                          2009042089

Printed in the United States of America by Hamilton Printing Company.

I would like to dedicate this book to the bedside nurse—whether a new graduate or a long-time dedicated professional who seeks to achieve excellence in nursing practice or to further educational goals by completing an advanced nursing degree. This is for you.

Contents

Preface

As a practicing nurse, I realize every day the importance of using the best evidence to deliver excellent and quality care to my patients. As an educator, I assist nurses to achieve their goal of obtaining their BSNs. While teaching a course entitled Evidence-Based Nursing Practice, I discovered that many of my students had never taken a basic research course. Indeed, they were fearful of research. I also had difficulty finding a suitable textbook that was written at the appropriate level and clearly explained the sometimes complex topics involved in research.

As a result, I decided to write my own book—one that nurses could use to understand basic research concepts, to assist them in obtaining "evidence" about their current daily practice, and to help them develop evidence-based practice (EBP) projects.

Therefore, this book aims to assist the experienced bedside nurse and recent graduate in understanding EBP and to embrace its implementation as a means of improving the quality of patient care. For the bedside nurse who may have significant clinical experience but may not have had the opportunity to take a research course, this book can serve as a guide to understanding the language and process of research. Alternatively, for the new nurse graduate, who may have taken a research course but may not have significant clinical experience, this book will serve as a useful reference in the workplace.

The book reviews the process of EBP, which involves defining a clinical situation of interest, formatting a good clinical question, conducting a literature search (i.e., finding the evidence), reading and critiquing research findings and/or published research reports, and deciding if the "evidence" warrants a change in practice. This book also reviews basic research terms and principles.

The newly qualified nurse researcher may find this book useful in implementing new research to create evidence when none is yet available. It is my hope that this book will empower the reader to become comfortable with research reports and the research process and to embrace and use research to suggest enhancements to the quality of patient care in the clinical environment.

This book is organized to assist bedside nurses in understanding and developing EBP projects that relate to their patient populations. This book delivers a wide scope of EBP content in an abbreviated style in the *Fast Facts* book series developed by Springer Publishing. Short chapters offer key content in a paragraph style using helpful headings and tables. Fast facts in a nutshell sections highlight important concepts and points in every chapter. Basic coverage of quantitative and qualitative research approaches are presented, as is an overview of EBP. This includes coming up with the "compelling question," finding and critiquing the evidence, and exploring the importance of disseminating what you have found to your colleagues and professionals throughout the world. This book also attempts to demystify systemic reviews and to explain how to conduct database searches. This book has been classroom tested and used in both live and on-line course formats.

Acknowledgments

I would like to acknowledge the RN students in my EBP course, who were interested and excited about learning EBP, tested this book, and offered valuable feedback. Thanks also to Laura M. Struble, PhD, GNP, BC, Clinical Assistant Professor at the University of Michigan School of Nursing who reviewed the manuscript. I would also like to acknowledge Barbara Chernow and Brian O'Connor for their assistance in refining and improving this project. I would also like to thank Margaret Zuccarini who has been a never-ending positive source of support in bringing my dream to a reality.

Chapter 1

Introduction to Evidence-Based Practice

INTRODUCTION

Every day, nurses are on the front line of patient care. It is the nurse who first notices a change in patient status. It is the nurse who implements and then evaluates the effectiveness of interventions. Often, nurses wonder who determines how nursing is practiced or why procedures are performed a certain way. A nurse might think, "It would be so much better if we did this procedure a different way." Did you ever wonder how you might change or impact the way patient care is delivered?

If you have ever asked yourself such questions or wondered about practice issues, evidence-based practice (EBP) can be your roadmap to suggesting change in the way patient care is delivered. It is the nurse who provides direct care to the patient. Why shouldn't the nurse identify patient care problems and procedural issues, thereby recommending the consideration of changes in how patient care is delivered? Now is the time for you to learn how you might use EBP strategies in your patient care area, unit, or institution.

In this chapter, you will learn:

1. The history of EBP.
2. The definition of EBP.
3. How to use EBP.
4. An example of EBP
5. The requirements for EBP.
6. Controversies surrounding EBP.
7. A rating system for the hierarchy of evidence in EBP.
8. The limitations of EBP.

BRIEF HISTORY OF EVIDENCE-BASED PRACTICE

A cornerstone of the evidence-based movement was laid by Dr. Archie Cochrane, a British epidemiologist. Cochrane struggled with the efficacy of health care and challenged patients to pay only for care that was judged effective through proven methods (http://www.cochrane.org/resources/brochure.htm). In 1972, Cochrane published a landmark book, Effectiveness and Efficiency: Random Reflections on Health Services, that criticized the medical profession for not conducting rigorous reviews of research evidence, so that organizations and policy makers could reach valid decisions about health care. Cochrane strongly advocated determining preferred treatment and practice by using evidence from randomized clinical trials (RCTs). His support of the development of a system to systematically organize this information led to the creation of the Cochrane library (http://www.cochrane.org/resources/brochure.htm). In 1993, **the Cochrane Collaboration was established to sup-**

port international efforts to improve health care throughout the world. More than 11,000 people contribute to the collaboration. Cochrane reviews bring together research on the effects of health care and are considered the gold standard for determining the effectiveness of different interventions (Cochrane Collaboration, 2007).

Research Utilization and Nursing

During the 1980s, the field of nursing supported efforts to apply research findings to practice. This process, called **research utilization, uses some aspect of a study in a manner unrelated to the intent of the original research.** It may result in changing practice based only on the findings of a single research study (Barnsteiner & Prevost, 2002). **As research is conducted over time, evidence accumulates about a particular topic (Polit & Beck, 2008) that can be used to varying degrees of clinical practice. For example,** after reading a qualitative research article about "hope" in patients with long-term chronic illnesses, a nurse may be more aware of the importance of maintaining hope when working with these patients. As a result, the nurse may become **more aware of how his or her actions may affect the hope of the patient. By using research utilization, the nurse will change his or her actions based of the reading of this one research article.** This may have not even been the original intent of the research project. It is important to note that this example illustrates the nurse demonstrating a greater awareness of the care he or she delivers. A nurse would not change actual physical care of a patient without a change in an approved protocol, but a physician might.

The difference between research utilization and EBP is that **research utilization may base changes in practice on the results of one study, whereas EBP answers a clinical question based on an in-depth literature search** conducted to find all relevant current research evidence related to that problem. So, while research utilization was an important concept to nursing, the EBP movement has led to important changes in clinical actions and practice **as a result of collaboration among the disciplines.**

Evolution from Research Utilization to Evidence-Based Practice

Because evidence-based practice is broader than research utilization, nursing professionals began to actively explore the advantages of reviewing and analyzing all of the available evidence on a given topic or problem before taking steps to recommend a change in practice. Thus, **EBP represented a major paradigm shift for healthcare education and nursing practice.** As the profession of nursing has evolved, nurses have become better educated and more involved in critiquing research studies. The purpose of critiquing is to analyze a study for flaws, evidence of bias, or other variables that might have affected the results. Polit and Beck (2008) note that a skillful clinician can no longer rely only on experience or a repository of memorized information, but must now be adept in accessing, evaluating, synthesizing, and applying new research evidence.

Fast facts in a nutshell

When evaluating research studies, make sure the research study design is congruent with its purpose. Quite simply, does the research study examine what it says it is going to?

Translating Research into Practice

Translating research evidence into actual nursing practice is a challenging process. Some **resources are available to help implement EBP, including integrative reviews, systematic reviews, meta-analyses, and clinical practice guidelines.**

- **Integrative reviews** are scholarly papers that offer generalizations about substantive issues based on a set of relevant studies. They synthesize published studies and articles to find answers to questions of interest. They are frequently found in peer-reviewed professional publications (Mileham, 2009).
- A **systematic review** is a state-of-the-art summary of all the research information available at a given time on a particular subject. This is not a literature review, but a review of actual research studies. All items in a systematic review address a specific clinical question. Systematic reviews can be found online at the Joanna Briggs Institute (http://www .joannabriggs.edu.au/pubs/systematic_reviews.php) and the

Cochrane Collaboration Center (http://www.cochrane.org/resources/handbook/). It is important to consider the source of a systematic review, particularly the credentials of the individual conducting the review and the integrity of the sources searched.

- A **meta-analysis** is a combination of the results of studies into a measureable format that statistically estimates the effects of proposed interventions and then critically reviews them to minimize bias. It is different from an integrative review in that it includes works that are similar or identical, so that a statistical comparison can be made (Schmidt & Brown, 2009).

- **Clinical practice guidelines** (CPGs) are available to help guide your clinical practice. As with systematic reviews, they distill a large amount of evidence into a manageable and usable format. **Clinical practice guidelines are practice recommendations based on the latest and best medical evidence available. They** can be used to guide clinical practice **and clinical decision-making that affects the** diagnosis, treatment, prevention, or management of a particular medical issue or condition. This means balancing the benefit and risks of an EBP decision. Clinical practice guidelines usually are based on systematic reviews and give specific practice recommendations and prescriptions for evidence-based decision making (Polit & Beck, 2008. CPGs are developed to help guide clinical practice even when only limited evidence is available. As multiple guidelines are being developed for the same topic, use the same rigor to critically appraise them as you would a research article.

Fast facts in a nutshell

Sources of Clinical Practice Guidelines

Sources for CPGs include the National Guideline Clearinghouse (http://www.guideline.gov), the Registered Nurses Association of Ontario (http://www.rnao.org/bestpractices), the Canadian Medical Association (http://www.cma.ca/index.cfm/ci_id/88655/la_id/1.htm), and Translating Research into Practice (http://www.tripdatabase.com/index.html). There are also guides specific to such specialties as, for example, women's health and neonatal nursing

---

Evidence-based practice is based on a comprehensive review of research findings, which emphasize intervention, randomized clinical trials (the gold standard), an integration of statistical findings, and the making of critical decisions about the findings based on the strength of the evidence, the tools used in the studies, and the cost (Jennings, 2000; Jennings and Loan, 2001). There are basic steps involved in implementing EBP (see Table 1.1)

Fast facts in a nutshell

Question: Do you have to be a nurse researcher to understand and utilize EBP?

Answer: *No. Evidence-based practice can be used by the bedside nurse to understand EBP and to devise EBP projects of his or her own that may lead to recommendations for change in clinical practices.*

There are basic steps involved in implementing EBP (see Table 1.1)

TABLE 1.1.   Seven Steps of Evidence-Based
                    Practice

---

1. Ask or identify the important clinical question.
2. Collect the best and most pertinent evidence.
3. Critically analyze and rate the evidence.
4. Integrate the evidence with your own clinical expertise, patient knowledge, and patient values in making a practice decision or recommending a change.
5. Implement your practice change, if authorized.
6. Evaluate how the practice change has influenced or affected your practice area.
7. Disseminate and share this evidence with your peers and colleagues.

DEFINITION OF EVIDENCE-BASED PRACTICE

The definition of EBP varies in relation to the concepts included. A search of the literature reveals that most definitions include (1) a focus on either the patient or the practitioner or (2) the three components: research-based information, clinical expertise or practice, and patient care. Melnyk and Fineout-Overholt (2005) define EBP as an "approach that enables clinicians to provide the highest quality of care in meeting the multifaceted needs of patients and families" (p. 3). An article by Melnyk (2003) states that EBP is "a problem solving approach to clinical decision making that incorporates a search for the best and latest evidence, clinical expertise and assessment, and patient preference and values within a context of caring" (p. 149). Rutledge and Grant (2002) define EBP as "care that integrates best scientific evidence with clinical expertise, knowledge of pathophysiology, knowledge of psychosocial issues, and decision making preferences of patients" (p. 1). This definition expands EBP to include consideration of pathophysiology and psychosocial issues in the decision-making process. Magee (2005) directs the definition toward physician care versus nursing care and states that EBP is "the conscientious, explicit, and judicious use of current best evidence in making decisions about the care of the individual patients" (p. 73). Pravikoff and coworkers offer a simplified definition of EBP as "a systematic approach to problem solving for healthcare providers, including RNs, characterized by the use of the best evidence currently available for clinical decision-making in order to provide the most consistent and best possible care to patients" (Pravikoff, Tanner, & Pierce, 2005, p.40). Ingersoll (2000) includes both the patient and the practitioner in her definition, as she defines EBP as "the conscientious, explicit, and judicious use of theory-driven research-based information in making decisions about care delivery to individuals or groups of patients and considers individual needs and preferences" (p.152).

After considering these definitions, how can we define EBP for nursing? Quite simply, **EBP is using the best available evidence to guide clinical practice so that patients receive the best possible nursing care.** It is important to differentiate among the terms evidence-based practice, evidence-based medicine, and evidence-based nursing, as they should not be used interchangeably. Evidence-based medicine is how physicians practice medicine. Evidence-based practice refers to physicians' or a nurses' use of evidence to guide practice. Finally, evidence-based nursing emphasizes nursing interventions that are based on the best evidence.

HOW DO I PARTICIPATE IN AN EVIDENCE-BASED PRACTICE?

Think of a clinical situation that generated questions in your mind for which you had no answers. There are several ways that you might try to find an answer to your question(s), including:

- Ask an authority or expert in the field.
- Consult a textbook.
- Look for an article in a nursing journal.
- Look for an article in a scholarly journal.
- Ask a nursing peer.
- Use simple trial and error.
- Use your intuition, judgment, or reasoning skills to solve the problem yourself.

As you can see, these responses are varied. In nursing, especially if time is critical, nurses may be required to make the best judgment at that moment. But, is this best practice? In making such a decision, does the nurse act in a routine manner in following accepted practice, or rather than as an individual who takes the steps to find answers to questions and thereby promote the knowledge base of nursing? **By using research evidence to guide practice, nurses can provide patients with the best interventions possible based on current research.**

Evidence-based practice uses current research findings as the basis for practice rather than using "acceptable standards" of practice. In essence, the latter meant doing things because "that is how we have always done them." Nurses may make specific decisions in caring for patients because they have been taught that the expert nurses' experience "works the best." Those expert experiences are important and valued, but they now are considered evidence that needs to be substantiated or validated through research and research dissemination in professional, scholarly, academic, and peer-reviewed publications. As the amount of evidence increases, so will EBP increase across professional nursing.

AN EXAMPLE OF EBP IN ACTION: SALINE VERSUS HEPARIN FLUSHES

Numerous studies have examined whether intermittent intravenous infusion reservoirs (heplocks or hepwells) remain as patent with flushes of normal saline solution as with use of a heparin lock solution. Research evidence has demonstrated that saline flushes are as effective as heparin flushes for maintaining peripheral intermittent infusion devices using larger than 24-gauge catheters. This has been studied frequently in children (Wong, 2002). Lombardi et al. (1988) conducted a sequential, nonrandom design of 74 catheter sites and found no difference in patency of catheters sized 20 to 24 gauge. In fact, there was a tendency for phlebitis to develop more often (13 versus 7 in the normal saline group) when using heparin flush solutions. Danek and Norris (2002) examined 160 infusion devices and found no difference in patency of 22 gauge catheters. These findings were also supported by McMullen et al. (1993), Hanrahan, Kleiber, and Fagen (1994), and Robertson (1994). Beecroft et al. (1997) did a collaborative study involving 9 hospitals and 451 subjects and found that heparin (10 units/ml and 100 units/ml) maintained catheters (sized 22 and 24 gauge) remained patent longer than did catheters that used saline alone as a flush. A randomized controlled trial by, Mok, Kwon, and Chan (2007), two of whom are clinical nurses and one a nursing professor, found no significant difference in the longevity of catheter patency or incidence of intravenous complications of 123 intravenous locks maintained with either saline flush, heparin flush (1 units/ml), and heparin flush (10 units/ml).

Now if you ask who first questioned the practice of using heparin flushes or if saline flushes might be as effective, you will learn that it was a nurse. This is just one example of how a nurse's observations and subsequent questioning changed nursing practice. Your observations or ideas, too, can change practice by initiating the question, conducting a literature review based on that question, examining the evidence and, if no evidence exists, suggesting that research studies might be needed to create the evidence to substantiate your hunches or ideas.

Fast facts in a nutshell

As a nurse embarking on EBP, it is important for you to first understand the basic concepts of research and how to rate or evaluate the evidence before suggesting that it be used to guide practice. Understanding nursing research will enable you to better apply research findings in your everyday practice.

REQUIREMENTS FOR AN EVIDENCE-BASED PRACTICE STUDY

The move toward EBP means, by definition, that **anyone can** conduct an exhaustive search of the literature and analyze the findings to determine the best evidence. **A hospital librarian or nursing colleague can assist you in getting started to find research articles.** A novice, who does not have the background or perhaps does not understand basic research methods, should ask a more experienced mentor for assistance in evaluating such research. Always remember that an EBP project requires an exhaustive, systematic, and analytical review of the literature. While one study should never result in a change in practice, the results of one study might provide the impetus to look at a current clinical process, construct a clinical question, and conduct further research that might support or invalidate the findings of that one study.

Fast facts in a nutshell

One research study should never change nursing clinical practice. A researcher must collect and analyze a complete review of the literature and then determine if this evidence has merit and should actually change practice.

The seasoned nurse must use sound reasoning and clinical judgment. Benner, Tanner, and Chesla (2009) describe clinical judgment as the way in which nurses come to understand and respond in concerned and involved ways based on salient information in a situation. Clinical judgment should encourage use of all types of available knowledge on which decisions can be based. The nurse's knowledge of patients or clients as people takes into consideration both cultural and ethical values in every step of the nursing process (Benner et al, 2009). For example, while research might show that a particular intervention is effective in reducing complications of stroke, this same intervention might not be acceptable in populations whose religious or cultural beliefs oppose this type of intervention.

CONTROVERSIES SURROUNDING EBP

Evidence-Based Practice as a "Cookbook Approach" to Care

One controversy about EBP is that it offers a "cookbook" approach to care and may override the individualization of care. Clinical decisions should be based on the evidence, as well as on a response to specific clinical situations or patients (Melnyk & Fineout-Overholt, 2005). It could also be argued that EBP might discourage attention to cultural issues, but nursing care must consider cultural variations in every given situation.

No Evidence

Another important controversy surrounding EBP is that no evidence may exist pertaining to a particular clinical question or that the "evidence" or research published on the clinical topic of interest is weak, poorly structured, or flawed. Another concern may be that existing evidence is too limited as a base for changing practice. For some topics of interest, there may be just one published research study. While you may be excited to find research on your topic of interest, it is important to critically evaluate the research that you have found. How do you conduct a critical evaluation to determine if it is good research? There are protocols to follow when evaluating research. If the research is not considered 'good' or reliable, then there is a need for a research study to be conducted on your clinical question, so that "good evidence" can be generated and published.

Randomized Clinical Trials

Some experts argue that a randomized clinical trial (RCT) is the gold standard for evaluating EBP results and other research methods should essentially be ignored. For example, qualitative research studies may yield valid and important evidence in exploring the problem under consideration, but may be disregarded in place of an RCT. The integration of the evidence for nursing practice is a key component for EBP. Nurses must pay attention to all types and levels of evidence and not simply look for or use RCTs, even though they are considered to be the highest level of evidence. In addition, the prudent nurse researcher should consider evidence from all disciplines, as well as all types of research methodology, to gain a thorough understanding of the available literature on the clinical question. The hierarchy and rating system for evaluating research evidence is provided in Table 1-2.

Finally it might be argued that EBP does not consider nursing theory as well as humanistic aspects of care. For those interested in nursing theory, very few research studies are based on or use nursing theory. This is another issue and concern voiced by the nursing profession.

LIMITATIONS OF EBP

Evidence-based practice faces limitations. Often, there is a shortage of good, coherent, and consistent scientific evidence in support of nursing practice. There is also difficulty in applying the evidence obtained to individual patients in partic-

TABLE 1.2.	Rating System for Hierarchy of Evidence

Level 1: Evidence from a systematic review or meta-analysis of all relevant RCTs or established EBP clinical guidelines.

Level 2: Evidence obtained from at least one well-designed RCT.

Level 3: Evidence obtained from a well-designed controlled trial without randomization or a systematic review of correlational/observational studies.

Level 4: Evidence from well-designed case-control and cohort studies that are correlational or observational.

Level 5: Evidence from systematic reviews of descriptive, qualitative, or physiologic studies.

Level 6: Evidence from a single descriptive, qualitative, or physiologic study.

Level 7: Evidence from the opinion of authorities/experts and/or case reports of expert committees.

Adapted from Polit & Beck (2008); Melnyk & Fineout-Overholt (2005).

ular clinical situations (Fain, 2009). Some nurses are hesitant or might even refuse to consider using EBP in their nursing practice and care. It is important to understand why this occurs. The reasons nurses give for not using research findings in their clinical practices are listed in Table 1.3.

TABLE 1.3.   Reasons Why Nurses Do Not Use Research Findings in Their Practices

1. Nurses may not know or be aware of research findings.
2. Nurses in practice do not usually associate or communicate with those who produce research findings.
3. Nurses lack the ability to locate and find relevant research reports.
4. Research is often in language that is not clinically meaningful.
5. Nurses do not understand research methods and have never had formal research classes in their nursing schools.
6. Nurses lack the value for research in practice.
7. Computer databases are not readily accessible to the nurse.
8. Nurses lack the basic knowledge to use information technology.
9. Nurses have no time to obtain this information.
10. Nurses do not understand exactly what evidence-based practice is.
11. People have a fear of the unknown and a fear of change. By understanding these processes, fear can be alleviated.

Table results adapted from Fain (2009) and Pravikoff, Tanner, & Pierce (2005)

Fast facts in a nutshell

A research study by Pravikoff, Tanner, and Pierce (2005) "Readiness of U.S. Nurses for Evidence-Based Practice," randomly sampled 3,000 nurses in the United States.

> The study concluded that while RNs generally acknowl-
> edge the need for information for effective practice, they
> simply were not prepared to use the information re-
> sources available to them.

The reasons why RNs were generally unprepared for EBP
include:

- limited time availability
- little or no education or training in information retrieval or
  accessing computer databases
- lack of needed basic computer skills
- limited access to high-quality information resources or databases
- attitudes that did not value or understand research.

Pravikoff et al. (2005) felt this could be attributed to the rapid
technological changes over the last 10 to 15 years, along with
the failure of nursing education programs to prepare students
at all levels to understand and value research-based practice
versus a practice based on tradition, intuition, and nursing
experience.

Once you have explored the beginnings of an EBP project
in the next few chapters, you will then learn why it is important to pay careful attention to overcoming the barriers to implementing EBP. Methods and suggestions will be discussed
in detail in Chapter 8.

Fast facts in a nutshell: summary

So, now is the time for you to learn about basic research principles and to increase your understanding of what evidence-based practice is all about. This book will guide you in unlocking the mysteries of EBP and help you understand how evidence can be used in your clinical area to change or improve practice. Let's get started by determining how EBP can be used by working through some examples of how an evidence-based project might begin.

REFERENCES

Barnsteiner, J., & Prevost, S. (2002). How to implement evidence-based practice. Some tried and true pointers. Reflections on Nursing Leadership, 28(2), 18–21

Beecroft, P.C., Bossert, E., & Chung, K. (1997). Intravenous lock patency in children: dilute heparin versus saline. Journal of Pediatric Pharmacology Practice, 2(4):211–223.

Benner, P., Tanner, C. A., & Chesla, C. A. (2009). Expertise in nursing practice: Caring, clinical judgment and ethics (2nd ed.). New York: Springer.

Cochrane, A. (1972). Effectiveness and efficiency: Random reflections on health care. London: Nuffield Provincial Hospitals Trust.

Cochrane Collaboration (2001). Retrieved July 20, 2007 from http://www.cochrane.org/resources/brochure.htm

Danek, G. D., & Noris, E. M. (1992). Pediatric IV catheters: efficacy of saline flush. Pediatric Nursing, 18(2):111–113.

Fain, J. A. (2009). Reading, understanding, and applying nursing research (3rd ed.). Philadelphia: F.A. Davis.

Hanrahan, K. S., Kleiber, C., & Fagan, C. (1994). Evaluation of saline for IV locks in Children. Pediatric Nursing, 20(6): 549–552.

Ingersoll, G. L. (2000). Evidence-based nursing: What it is and what it isn't. Nursing Outlook, 48, 151–152.

Jennings, B. W. (2000). Evidence-based practice: The road best traveled? Research in Nursing and Health, 23(5), 343–345.

Jennings, B. W., & Loan, L. A. (2001). Misconceptions among nurses about evidence-based practice. Journal of Nursing Scholarship, 33(2), 121–127.

Lohr, K. N. Eleazer, K., & Mauskopf, J. (1998). Health policy issues and applications for evidence-based medicine and clinical practice guidelines. Health Policy, 46, 1–19.

Lombardi T. P., et al. (1988). Efficacy of 0.9% sodium chloride injection with or without heparin sodium for maintaining patency of intravenous catheters in children, Clinical Pharmacology, 7(11):832–836.

Magee, M. (2005). Health politics: Power, population and health. Bronxville, NY: Spencer Books.

McMullen, A., et al. (1993). Heparinized saline or normal saline as a flush solution in intermittent intravenous lines in infants and children, American Journal of Maternal/Child Nursing, 18(2):78–85.

Melnyk, B. M. (2003). Finding and appraising systematic reviews of clinical interventions: Critical skills for evidence-based practice. Journal of Pediatric Nursing, 29(2), 147–149.

Melnyk, B. M., & Fineout-Overholt, E. (2005) Evidence-based practice in nursing and health care: A guide to best practice. Philadelphia: Lippincott, Williams & Wilkins.

Mileham, P. (2009). Finding sources of evidence. In N. Schmidt & J. Brown (Eds.), Evidence-based practice: Appraisal and applications of research. Boston: Jones & Barlett.

Mok, E., Kwon, T, & Chan, M. F. (2007). A randomized controlled trial for maintaining peripheral intravenous infusion devices in children. International Journal of Nursing Practice, 13(1), 33–45.

National Guideline Clearinghouse. (2009). Retrieved July 3, 2009 from http://www.guideline.gov/index.aspx

Polit, D. F., & Beck, C. T. (2008). Nursing research: Generating and assessing evidence for Nursing Practice (8th Ed.). Philadelphia: Lippincott, Williams, & Wilkins.

Pravikoff, D. S., Tanner, A. B., & Pierce, S. T. (2005). Readiness of U.S. nurses for evidence-based practice. American Journal of Nursing, 105(9), 40–51.

Robertson J. (1994). Intermittent intravenous therapy: a comparison of two flushing solutions, Contemporary Nursing, 3(4):174–179.

Rutledge, D. N., & Grant, M. (2002). Introduction. Seminars in Oncology Nursing, 18, 1–2.

Schmidt, N. A., & Brown, J. M. (2009). Evidence-based practice for nurses: Appraisal and application of research. Sudbury, MA: Jones & Bartlett.

Wong, D. (2002). Saline Versus Heparin Flush for Peripheral Intermittent IV Infusions in Children. Available on-line at http://www.mosbysdrugconsult.com/WOW/p049.html

Chapter 2

Asking the Compelling Question

INTRODUCTION

When beginning an evidence-based practice (EBP) project, several steps are crucial to consider, including developing a well-constructed clinical question. Taking time to construct a clinical question is of chief importance because this question will drive every aspect of your research, from the initial literature search to the final success of your project. This chapter explains how to begin selecting your clinical question and provides tools to construct a high-quality clinical question.

In this chapter, you will learn:

1. How to start an evidence-based practice project.
2. How to structure a compelling clinical question.
3. How to use the PICO model in implementing evidence based practice.
4. How to determine if a study is valid and reliable.

HOW TO START AN EVIDENCE-BASED PRACTICE PROJECT

Sackett, Richardson, Rosenberg, and Hayes (2000) described this step as the most challenging in the EBP process. Where do you find an appropriate question? **Your clinical or work environment presents many opportunities for developing a compelling question**, such as these listed below.

1. Has there been a time in clinical practice when you have wondered, "Why do we do it this way" and, after asking a colleague, receive the answer, "because that is the way we have always done it" or "because that is the only way it works?" The next time you hear these words, take a step back and ask yourself, "Does this make sense?"
2. Why do nurses always use a black pen to chart their notes? Is it simply preference or the result of trial and error? The reason is simple. When photocopying and scanning notes into the computer database, black ink shows up better than blue. This illustrates a trial-and-error method of problem solving, but it also provides a relevant example of a possible source of a compelling clinical question.
3. Have you wondered why bed alarms are used for particular patients? The answer is that a research study showed that bed alarms decreased the number of patient falls on a given unit. A screening tool identified patients considered to be "at risk." For these patients, a bed alarm was activated, and the fall risk for those patients was reduced. This sounds quite basic, but several research studies have shown the effectiveness of bed alarms in decreasing pa-

tient falls. This nursing practice is a good example of evidence-based practice.

Other areas to consider when searching for a compelling clinical question include etiology, diagnoses, therapies, prevention strategies, and prognoses. Questions you might consider are those that provide meaning or insight into a phenomenon that might help nurses to appreciate or relate to a patient's experience or to understand the growing impact of culture on the administration of healthcare today. With the skyrocketing cost of health care, the question could also include a cost-containment measure or an intervention that could decrease the length of a patient's stay in the hospital. All of these are areas for an inquisitive mind to explore.

Current research studies usually conclude with a summary discussion and a section describing the implications for further research. These are both potential sources of ideas for clinical questions. Thus, if you have the experience and qualifications, your initial EBP project may enable you to design and conduct your own research study. It is perfectly acceptable to build on existing research and answer a question posed by another author. This can be a **research problem** that is an area of concern or that illustrates a gap in current knowledge or in the literature. This research problem can also be the impetus to helping to form your EBP clinical question.

In developing an EBP project, one could also consider questions that might build on current nursing theory. Investigate national initiatives by U.S. government agencies, some of which routinely identify health problems and sometimes suggest research priorities. Topical areas suggested by authors for further investigation do not necessarily have to develop into full research studies, but they can inspire an EBP project. This is particularly true if it proves to be an area that might save a healthcare agency money or improve a process. Some excellent places to start might be the research agendas for health concerns (Adams, 2009), examples of which are available on the following government Web sites:

- The U.S. Surgeon General's Office. (http://www.surgeongeneral.gov/)
- The National Institute of Health (http://www.nih.gov)
- The National Institute of Nursing Research (http://www.ninr.nih.gov/)
- The National Institute of Mental Health (http://www.nimh.nih.gov/)

Who knows? Your EBP project could develop into a research study.

The clinical question you develop will most likely fall into one of the following categories:

- Diagnosis identification or recognition.
- Therapy or intervention.
- Etiology.
- Impact of the prognosis.
- Prevention strategy.

HOW TO STRUCTURE THE COMPELLING QUESTION IN A SEARCHABLE AND ANSWERABLE FORMAT

When asking a compelling question, be sure the question is phrased so that it can be answered. If worded too broadly, you may not be able to find a usable answer. Simply restating the question may sometimes solve this problem. For example, perhaps you wanted to ask, "Why are patients angry?" Although this is a good question, it really is too broad to answer meaningfully or specifically. A better question would be, "Are anger levels lower in patients admitted to the emergency room as compared to patients admitted directly to the medical surgical floor?" Note that you have narrowed your focus a comparison between anger levels in patients being admitted to two different units. This is much more specific. The environment in which they are may or may not play a part in their anger. The more specific your question, the more answerable it becomes.

Another consideration is the amount of evidence available to answer your question. If a lot of evidence exists, your question may already have been asked multiple times and does not need to be asked again. If this might be the situation in relation to your question, move on to another question. On the other hand, if no evidence is available to support your question, you may have an important question that should be explored. Where will you begin to find the evidence to support a question that has never been asked? First, you might look to the field of medicine for relevant studies and then to related disciplines.

For example, you might decide to investigate the stress a family member experiences when walking into the intensive care unit for the first time. If you can find no nursing studies on this topic, you should look at resources in psychology that explore stress and coping theory. While these studies may not have been conducted in the intensive care environment, they relate by focusing on the human reaction to stress.

THE PICO FORMAT

Many methods are available for implementing EBP projects. One simple method used in this book is the PICO format, presented by Melnyk and Fineout-Overholt (2005).

Fast facts in a nutshell

The PICO acronym is broken down as follows:
   P = Patient population of interest
   I = Intervention of interest
   C = Comparison of interest
   O = Outcome of interest

Step One: Defining the Patient Population of Interest

The first step in coming up with a research or evidence-based practice question is to decide what **population** you want to examine. Are you interested in infants, children, adults, or geriatric individuals? Perhaps you are interested in people with psychological disorders or people with whom you deal in the community. In defining the population, describe the group clearly. If you are interested in studying the geriatric or "elderly" group, does what ages will you include in your group: people over the age of 50, 55, 60, or 65? Will your group include male or female patients, or both? If you are interested in working with "children," what ages will you include in your group: infants, toddlers, preschoolers, school-age children, or adolescents? Will your group include boys or girls, or both? Be very clear when defining your population of interest.

The reason the patient population must be carefully described is that you want the search engines to give you relevant information and not information that is too broad or off target. When retrieving information in a literature search, keep in mind that research findings of one patient population may not be relevant to another (Adams, 2009). For example, if you are looking at the effects of thrombolytic agents in children, and you find a study that examines thrombolytic agents in adults, you cannot assume that the thrombolytic agent will work the same in different patient populations. This is only one of many important variables to consider that can affect any study.

Fast facts in a nutshell

When looking at a certain population, be sure to consider age, gender, race, ethnicity, disease process or comorbidities, or any characteristic that may affect the chosen population of interest.

Step Two: Identifying the Intervention or Process of Interest

The second step is to decide what **intervention** or **process** you want to examine. What do you want to do for this patient population? Ask yourself these questions:

- Have you ever asked why nurses follow a particular process and never received a logical answer?
- Have I found that performing an intervention in one particular way seems to be more effective than another?
- Have I seen patients improve and recover more quickly when a particular intervention has been used?
- Have I noticed that when a particular physician is on call, the patients do better—or worse—in relation to a particular intervention?
- Have I noticed that the unit seems to have a large number of infected central lines, or sepsis?
- Have I noticed that the unit seems to be calmer when certain individuals are working and less controlled when other individuals are present? Why? Is there something different in the care delivered?
- Have I noticed that there might be a better and more cost-effective way to perform an intervention I do every day?
- Do I feel that practice standards in a particular area are lacking?
- Have I recently read an article about a particular topic and thought, "Hey, that is a good idea" or "Why do we not do that in my unit?"

These are just some questions that could be the impetus for finding a better way or to justify a existing way that nursing practice and interventions are performed. Quite simply, ask yourself what is the burning question or pet peeve of yours that just does not make sense in performing your daily nursing routine? What do you feel could be done better? Is there something you feel is wasteful and could be done a different way to decrease costs, improve patient outcomes, or reduce time required? Table 2.1 contains information to consider when looking at each of these questions.

In researching an intervention or treatment, remember to compare the reaction of the individual who receives the intervention with the reaction of the individual who does not receive the treatment. If the latter group received a placebo, the effect of that placebo must also be considered. Patients who receive a placebo, or harmless intervention, think they have received the actual treatment. As such, they constitute a control group against which the patients receiving the actual intervention can be measured. If, for example, the subjects who received the sugar pill experience any "effects," they are known as "placebo effects." The more defined the intervention, the more focused your question will be, so that it will avoid any placebo effects.

Step Three: Examining the Comparison of Interest

The comparison of interest is the alternative to your intervention. The comparison can be **a control (no treatment) versus a placebo (fake treatment)**. The comparison can also consist of **measuring your intervention of interest against what is considered the "gold standard"** of treatment for a particular situation or disease process. For example, you might plan to use a fall intervention strategy with the elderly population.

TABLE 2-1. The PICO Method	
Patient population of interest	The patient population for the problem of interest: • Age • Gender • Ethnicity • Educational status • With certain disease process or disorder (i.e. heart disease, diabetes, pancreatitis)
Intervention	The intervention or interventions of interest • Exposure to disease • Prognostic factor A • Risk behaviors (i.e. smoking, drug usage, cholesterol levels)
Comparison	What you want to compare the intervention to or against • No disease • Placebo or no intervention • Type of therapy given or not • Prognostic factor B • Absence of a risk factor or characteristic (i.e. a non-smoker, non-drug user)
Outcome	Outcome of interest, what is the result? • Risk of disease • Accuracy of diagnosis • Rate of occurrence of adverse outcome (i.e. severe illness, development of a co-morbidity, or even death)

Table adapted from Melnyk and Fineout-Overholt (2005).

First, you learn what the literature says about fall intervention in your patient population. Then, you conduct a minisurvey of your patient population and fall interventions. Finally, compare your fall intervention strategy group to a group of elderly patients who do not receive that specific intervention. You could also do a simple performance improvement (PI) or quality assurance (QA) survey of your patient population. This does not have to involve a large group. You can then compare what you found in the literature with what you found on your unit. This data can be impressive when approaching the administration to consider implementing a practice change. Such a survey is not necessary; you could just present the evidence. But, including survey data from your institution's patient population in addition to the review of the literature will result in a stronger presentation.

Another example is the use of pain medication in the pediatric population. One group could receive a narcotic medication in the form of a lollipop (i.e. Fentanyl lollipops), while the other group does not. The comparison of interest would be an evaluation of any difference in the level of pain experienced by the two groups. Again, you would search the literature first and then conduct an informal survey of your patients. Keep in mind which patients are receiving such medications and which patients are undergoing which procedures. As this may go beyond a simple survey of your patient population, it may require administrative and institutional review board (IRB) approval. Always check with your hospital administration before embarking on any type of data collection procedures to be sure you are operating within institutional policy and always maintaining patient confidentiality.

To make an adjustment to the above example to compare the type of intervention, consider if one group of children received the narcotic lollipop and another group received a a regular lollipop without medication in it. The comparison of interest would be if the groups experienced different levels of pain. In this example, you would need to use the same developmentally appropriate pain scale to measure pain in both groups. This would be a 0 to 10 scale for older adolescent children and, perhaps, the faces scale for school-aged children.

Step Four: Outcome of Interest

The last step is establishing the outcome of interest. What will be improved or what do you want to see happen to the patient? **What do you want to accomplish or measure?** The Cochrane Collaboration *Handbook* (2008) notes that the outcome of your study should be important and not trivial. Include outcomes that might be meaningful to the people who make decisions about healthcare practice. For example suppose you researched whether adults who received supplemental feedings have an improved outcome of gaining weight. You would ask the question, "Do fragile geriatric individuals aged 65 and older gain weight when provided with supplemental calorie shakes with meals?" Your outcome will be gaining weight. By specifically stating your outcome in your question, you will more accurately focus the search for evidence in the literature. As a result, you will find more relevant studies than if you searched for "protein shakes" alone.

> ## Fast facts in a nutshell
>
> The University of Alberta, Canada, Libraries provides a free download of its PICO maker Palm OS-based software at obtained from its Web site at http://www.library.ualberta.ca/pdazone/pico/

Recommended Step Five: Time Frame

Fineout-Overholt and Johnston (2005) have recommended adding a fifth element to the PICO method, making it the PICOT method. The last component "T" stands for time; the time frame in which the question occurs. While it is helpful to establish a timeline for completion of the PICO process, parts of the process may be out of your control. Still, establishing deadlines will help you stay focused and on task.

Schlosser and Costello (2007) propose the PESICO method, which stands for person, environment, stakeholders, intervention, comparison, and outcome. These authors believe that environment should be included as it can directly affect the outcome, and that one must establish which of the stakeholders in a study stand to gain or lose? These important sources of influence need to be considered when undertaking an EBP project.

EVALUATING VALIDITY AND RELIABILITY

When examining research studies, **consider if the study is reliable and valid**. These two terms should be understood and applied to your EBP project.

- **Validity** is the ability to measure what it is supposed to or is intended to be measured.
- **Reliability** is the ability to measure what you want to measure on subsequent experiences.

If your institution is purchasing new blood glucose meters, the meters should be tested to ensure that they accurately measure blood glucose levels every time (validity). The meters should measure the blood sugar of 100 the same way each time it performs a test on a patient (reliability). **To be valid and reliable, the meters should consistently meet these criteria.** These are also the reasons why if you come across a nonfunctional piece of equipment in your clinical environment, you should remove it immediately from service. These terms will be explored more in Chapter 7, Evaluating the Evidence.

The following five cases are designed to help define and focus your clinical question using the PICO method.

CASE STUDIES

CASE STUDY 2.1

You work in a pediatric unit at a local hospital. Children are being readmitted for rotavirus, which is a gastrointestinal illness that results in severe diarrhea and abdominal cramping. The children frequently present with severe dehydration. The virus is transmitted through contact via the fecal-oral route. Each of these children was in the hospital a week prior to this second admission for another illness. As you think about this, you realize that these children must be getting this infection nosocomially. You suspect hand washing may be a problem on your unit. You want to explore this occurrence through an EBP study. Fill in the blanks for the potential question of interest.

Does the *incidence of readmission* to the pediatric floor of
_____ (P) ___ _____ patients decrease when proper *hand washing is demonstrated by healthcare personnel* as compared to
_____ (C) _____ their hands?

Where,
P = pediatric patients aged < 8
I = washing their hands
C = washing hands versus not washing hands
O = incidence (or decrease) in the readmission of patients.

Answer: (P) = pediatric patients <8 years of age; (C) = not washing their hands

CASE STUDY 2.2

You work in a busy emergency department in a level-one trauma center. You notice an increase in the number of young adult patients admitted with severe head injury. Your state has just changed the law so that motorcycle riders are not required to wear helmets. Fill in the blanks below.

Does wearing _____ (I) _____ *verses not wearing a helmet* while riding a motorcycle decrease the *amount of admissions to the ED* for severe head injury _____ (P) _____ ?

Where,
P = young adult patients aged < 25
I   = wearing a helmet
C = wearing or not wearing a helmet
O = decrease the admission of motorcycle riders

Answer: (I) = a helmet; (P) = in young adult patients aged <25 years old

CASE STUDY 2.3

A 78-year-old man comes into the doctor's office for a regular check up. His blood pressure is 160/98. His physical exam is otherwise normal. He is normally on blood pressure medication. When asked if he takes his medication regularly, he says yes and mentions that he also takes a multivitamin and some "natural remedies." He lives alone and is independent in all of his activities of daily living. His daughter, who visits him weekly, is with him for the appointment.

(continued)

You ask both of them if you can do anything to assist him in "remembering" to take his medication. You consult the literature and find out 75% of elderly individuals living alone forget to take their medications on a daily basis.

Does _____ (I) _____ medications for _____ (P) _____ improve their *compliance in taking their oral medications and maintain a stable blood pressure* than those who do *not get their oral medications poured for them each week?*

Where,
P = Elderly individuals > age 70 living alone
I = Compliance with taking medications by placing them weekly in a plastic container marked with the days of the week and times of the day.
C = Elderly people using the "prepouring' method, and elderly people not using this method.
O = Those who have their medications poured weekly for them will have an increased compliance of taking their medications and maintaining stable blood pressure.

Answer: (I) = placing medications in a plastic box marked with the days of the week.; (P) = elderly patients aged >70 years of age living alone.

CASE STUDY 2.4

You work in a rural hospital in the labor and delivery department. Within the last six months, you notice that the new Certified Nurse Anesthetist (CNA) and physicians have started offering epidural anesthesia for all routine vaginal deliveries. You note that of the last
(continued)

100 vaginal deliveries, 89 had epidural anesthesia. You wonder if this is necessary or presented as a choice to the mother. You decide to consult the literature looking for evidence.

Does _____ (I) _____ anesthesia for _____ (P) _____ as *compared to a natural delivery method affect the level of noncomplicated delivery?*

Where,
P = laboring vaginal delivery patients
I = epidural anesthesia
C = epidural anesthesia or no anesthesia and a natural delivery method
O = Decreased level of delivery patients without complications

Answer: (I) = epidural anesthesia; (P) = laboring vaginal delivery patients

---

CASE STUDY 2.5

You work in an adult intensive care burn unit. You notice standard protocol stipulates that tube feedings are usually not started until the fifth day of admission to the burn unit. You wonder why tube feedings are not started earlier and whether that increases or decreases the length of stay of these patients in the burn unit. You also wonder if they are getting the proper nutrition, as they are in a hypermetabolic state. What effect does this have on their weight and nutritional status? You consult the literature to find studies on the timing of feeding adult burn unit patients. The literature shows that tube feeding started in the first 24 hours of admission to the burn unit decreases the morbidity and length of stay in burn units across the country.

(continued)

Does *starting tube feedings* on day _____ (C^1) _____ verses day _____ (C^2) _____ *increase or decrease the length of stay* of the _____ (P) _____ *in the burn unit?*

Where,

P = adult burn patients >age 18 in the burn unit
I = starting tube feedings on day 1
C = starting tube feedings on day 1 versus day 5
O = increase in weight gain, increased nutrition, decrease in
length of stay.

In addition, you could also compare weight gain or loss for adult burn patients over 18 years of age depending on whether tube feedings start on day 1 or day 5.

Answer: (C^1) = day 1; (C^2) – day 5; (P) = adult burn patients >18 years of age.

Fast facts in a nutshell: summary

Once you select a topic for your EBP project, be specific in defining your patient population and environment. If your question is too broad, it may not be answerable or you may not find evidence on that particular subject. By narrowing your question and asking it in an answerable format, you will increase the ease of developing your EBP project. A key is to see how well your question fits into an EBP model, such as the PICO format.

REFERENCES

Adams, S. (2009). Indentifying research questions. In N. A. Schmidt & J. M. Brown (Eds.), *Evidence-based practice for nurses: Appraisal and application of research* (pp 57–74). Boston: Jones & Bartlett.

Cochrane Collaboration (2008). *Cochrane handbook for systematic reviews of interventions*. Retrieved June 9, 2009 from http://www.cochrane.org/resources/handbook/

Fineout-Overholt, E., & Johnston, L. (2005). Teaching EBP: Asking searchable, answerable clinical questions. *Worldviews on Evidence-Based Nursing, 2*(3), 157–160.

Melnyk, B. M., & Fineout-Overholt, E. (2005). *Evidence-based practice in nursing and healthcare: A guide to best practice.* Philadelphia: Lippincott, Williams & Wilkins.

Sackett, D., Richardson, W., Rosenberg, W., & Hayes, R. (2000). *Evidence-based medicine: How to practice and teach EBM.* New York: Churchill Livingstone.

Schlosser, R. W., Koul, R., & Costello, J. (2007). Asking well-built questions for evidence-based practice in augmentative and alternative communication. *Journal of Communication Disorders, 40*(3), 225–238.

Chapter 3

A Basic Understanding of Research

INTRODUCTION

You might think that now that you have decided on a compelling question, you are ready to search for evidence. But before beginning your evidence-based project (EBP), you need to understand some basic principles. That way, when you find "evidence," you will know what type it is; how to classify and interpret it; and whether the research finding constitutes "good evidence". This chapter provides an overview of the research process, as well as the proper terminology. For additional explanations about the process, consult a research text. Remember that you will not be conducting a research study. Rather, you will be conducting an evidence-based practice project.

In this chapter, you will learn:

1. A basic history of nursing research.
2. The two basic types of research.
3. The steps in the research process.

A HISTORY OF NURSING RESEARCH

When did nursing research begin? Florence Nightingale introduced the concept of scientific inquiry as the basis of nursing practice. She began collecting information and making observations about soldier mortality and morbidity during the Crimean War. With this scientific data, she fought for changes in nursing practice that affected outcomes for soldiers in the war (Houser, 2008). Her work to improve sanitary conditions in the 1800s was one of the first times a nurse linked environmental conditions (variables) to clinical or patient outcomes. Nightingale also kept detailed notes on her patients. Her book *Notes on Nursing* presents her initial observations and findings. **While Nightingale did not practice evidence-based research, her findings were based on her experience and observations.** While simplistic by today's methods, her approach reflects a rudimentary form of the nursing research process.

TWO BASIC CATEGORIES OF RESEARCH

The two **main categories of nursing research are quantitative and qualitative.** In quantitative studies, the researcher identifies variables of interest and collects relevant data from subjects. This data usually takes on a numerical format (Polit & Beck, 2010). For example, suppose the researcher is measuring happiness using a quantitative approach. The researcher would need to quantify happiness using a numeric happiness scale on which subjects could objectively quantify their level of happiness. This could be on a scale of 0 to 10 on a continuum, where 0 is no happiness and 10 is extreme happiness.

In qualitative studies, the researcher collects narrative data or descriptions by having conversations with the research participants, making observations, and taking notes. These interactions usually occur in the participants' natural environments, such as home, workplace, or a mutually agreed upon venue. Diaries may also be used (Polit & Beck, 2010). If the happiness study discussed above was a qualitative study, the researcher would ask participants to describe their happiness by asking a broad question, such as "tell me about your happiness," and paying careful attention not to persuade or influence the participants' answers.

See Table 3.1 for a comparison of qualitative and quantitative research on the question of pain. These research methods will be discussed in greater depth in Chapters 4 and 5.

Quantitative Research

Quantitative research is objective. It imposes tight control over the research situation. It generalizes findings and frequently includes numbers, facts, and figures. When you think of quantitative research think **numbers**. The study sample usually has a large number of participants or subjects.

Qualitative Research

Qualitative research is more subjective. It describes an individual's experience in the participant's own words. This narrative or verbal description is obtained after the researcher asks the participant an open-ended question and allows the participant to share his or her thoughts and feelings (see Chapter 5). Qualitative research usually has fewer participants in the sample than quantitative studies. Statistical analysis is used and common themes are sought and identified. For further clarification of this analysis, consult a basic research text.

TABLE 3.1 Example: PAIN	
Quantitative Study	Qualitative Study
Criterion: Numerical scale 0 to 10 Answer: "pain was 3 out of 10"	Criterion: verbal description, tell me more about your pain Answer: "the pain was crushing and the worst pain I ever had"

Fast facts in a nutshell

- Quantitative research is objective.
- Qualitative research is subjective.

TABLE 3.2   Steps in the Research Process

1. Identify the problem.
2. Determine the purpose of the study.
3. Determine the study variables.
4. Conduct a literature review.
5. Identify a theoretical or conceptual framework.
6. Identify study assumptions.
7. Formulate the hypothesis and/or research questions.
8. Identify the type of research design.

STEPS IN THE RESEARCH PROCESS

The following is a description of the steps in the research process (see also Table 3.2). Some may overlap, some can be varied, and some can be combined.

Step One: Identify the Problem (problem statement)

The first and perhaps the most important part of the research process is to clearly identify the problem. What is it that the researcher wants to study? This problem should be of interest to the researcher and should also be of significance to nursing. For example, a pediatric nurse may be interested in studying the best method of measuring temperature in a child, but the question is whether the conclusion would really make a difference to the field of nursing. A review of the literature reveals that this topic has been studied frequently, with 35 studies agreeing on the most accurate method. This topic clearly does not need to be studied again. Now, suppose that same nurse learns that a new device for temperature taking, such as a femoral thermometer, has just been invented. If the nurse wants to study if the femoral method is as accurate as the rectal method, this is a new and important question. By conducting this research study, one could determine if this new method is indeed accurate and, if so, if it should be recommended as the preferred method for use in pediatric units across the country.

The problem statement can be one declarative or interrogative sentence that includes a clear identification of the population to be studied and the variables involved. The last thing for the researcher to consider is if the problem is empirically testable. The problem statement is the "what" of the study. What is going to be examined by the researcher and can it be done?

Fast facts in a nutshell

Declarative statement:
Femoral thermometer readings are more accurate than the rectal method in pediatric patients from 1 to 4 years of age.

Interrogative statement:
Are femoral thermometers as accurate as rectal thermometers in pediatric patients from 1 to 4 years of age?

TABLE 3.3   Guidelines for Writing and Critiquing a Problem Statement

1. Is the problem statement clear and concise?
2. Is the problem statement written in a declarative or interrogatory sentence?
3. Are the study variables and population of interest included in the problem statement?
4. Does the problem statement indicate that the study would be feasible or able to be carried out?
5. Does the problem statement indicate that it is clinically significant or relevant to nursing practice?

Table adapted from Nieswiadomy (2008).

There are many things to consider when writing a good problem statement. See Table 3.3 for guidelines in writing and critiquing the problem statement.

Step Two: State the Purpose of the Study

This step defines the reason for the study? What is the purpose? **Why does one want to study this topic?** What is the goal, or aim? For example, the statement of purpose for the problem identified above, which involves methods of measuring temperature in pediatric patients, might read as follows, "The purpose of the study is to determine which method of measuring temperature in pediatric patients from 1 to 4 years of age is more accurate." Sometimes the problem statement and the purpose are seen as the same, but they really are not. The problem statement is the "what" of the study. It formally identifies the problem being addressed. It includes the scope of the research problem, the specific population being studied, the independent and dependent variables, and the goal or question the study is trying to answer (Gillis & Jackson, 2002). In comparison, the purpose of the study is the "why" of what is being examined, and it derives from the problem statement (Adams, 2009). Both statements should be mentioned near the beginning of the study.

Fast facts in a nutshell

Problem statements identify "what" the study is about; the purpose statement indentifies "why" the study is being conducted.

Step Three: Determine the Study Variables

In an experimental study, the concepts or items of interest to be studied are called variables. A variable is a something that can change. For example, weight, age, and body temperature are all variables that can be studied (Polit & Beck, 2008). **Variables can be independent or dependent.** An independent variable is the "cause" or the variable that influences the dependent variable. The **dependent variable** is the "effect," or that which is influenced by the independent variable. The dependent variable can also be called the **criterion** or **outcome variable**. It is the variable that is observed for change or reaction after the intervention has been applied (Fain, 2009). For examples of independent and dependent variables, see Table 3.4.

For example, if the researcher was looking at the relationship between age and the amount of exercise people do, the independent variable would be age and the dependent variable would be exercise. In this case, age is not the cause of the amount of exercise performed, but the direction of influence or the item or issue identified that influences the second vari-

---

TABLE 3.4   Examples of Independent Variables (IVs) and Dependent Variables (DVs)

---

1. Problem statement: "In the hospital, does the presence of a support group for head injured patients affect the stress level of patients with head injuries?"
   IV = presence of support group
   DV = stress level of patients

2. Problem statement: "Is there a difference between the development of breast cancer in women who eat meat and those who do not eat meat?"
   IV = those who eat meat and do not eat meat
   DV = development of breast cancer

3. Problem Statement: "Is there a difference in NCLEX test scores between baccalaureate nursing students and associate degree nursing students?"
   IV = BSN students and ADN students
   DV = test scores

---

able (exercise) (Nieswiadomy, 2008). It is clear from this example that age may have a direct influence on the amount of exercise a person is able to do. So this is another way that variables play an important role in the research process. For more on variables, see Chapter 4.

What, indeed, are the variables included in a study? There may be one, two, or many variables in a study. A one-variable study is also called a **univariate study**. An example of a problem statement with only one variable would be, "What are the sources of stress in the Emergency Department?" Here the researcher is only looking at one variable as the source of stress.

A two-variable study is also called a **bivariate study**. Usually, one variable is the independent variable and the second a dependent variable. An example of a bivariate study question is, "Does the speed of driving correlate to the incidence of automobile accidents in adolescents?" An automobile accident is the independent variable, and the speed of the car is the dependent variable. A second example of a bivariate study question is the interrogatory problem statement, "Does the level of stress affect final exam scores for senior BSN students?" The cause or level of stress in this case will have a direct effect of the final exam scores, which is the dependent variable. Table 3.5 offers examples of types of problem statements using variables.

Fast facts in a nutshell

An independent variable is the "cause" or the variable which influences the dependent variable. The dependent variable is the "effect" or that which is influenced by the independent variable.

TABLE 3.5 Variables in Problem Statement Format

Correlational Statement: Is there a correlation between X (independent variable) and Y (the dependent variable)?

Example: *Is there a correlation between the level of stress and final exam scores of nursing students?*

Comparative Statement: Is there a difference in Y (dependent variable) between people who have X (independent variable) and those who do not have X?

Example: *Is there a difference in stress levels of nursing students who attended a review course and those who did not?*

Experimental Study Statement: Is there a difference in Y (dependent variable) between people who received X (independent variable) and those who did not receive X (independent variable)?

Example: *Is there a difference in pain in pediatric patients who received EMLA cream and those who did not receive EMLA cream prior to venipuncture?*

There are other types of variables. **Extraneous variables,** for example, are those not under investigation or examination but still may or may not be relevant to, or interfere with, the study. Extraneous variables may be controlled or uncontrolled by the researcher. It is best for the researcher to try to identify any extraneous variables and control them, so that they will not interfere with the purpose of the experiment or result in any adverse or unplanned effects. Extraneous variables may also be called **confounding variables, intervening variables,** or **mediating variables** (Fain, 2009; LoBiondo-Wood, & Haber,

2006). An example of an extraneous variable occurs in the study of older men who are enrolled in a new exercise program (independent variable) to determine how exercise affects their lung condition (dependent variable) by measuring functional lung capacity. The extraneous variables that could affect the dependent variable would be age, a history of smoking (including the length of time and the amount the patient smoked), second-hand smoke exposure, and comorbid conditions, such as chronic obstructive pulmonary disorder (COPD), lung cancer, asthma, or any diagnosis that might affect the dependent variable of actual functional lung capacity. So, the researcher would be wise to address these issues by eliminating from the study men who had smoked and had a preexisting or comorbid condition of COPD and asthma.

Step Four: Conduct a Review of the Literature

The review of the literature can be an overwhelming task for the novice researcher. If one is experiencing difficulty conducting the literature review, consult a colleague or a librarian who is experienced with the process of finding research articles. They are excellent resources and usually are willing to help.

Research in any field must build on what already has been done. Therefore, **nurse researchers must locate relevant studies about the problem of interest to determine where the gaps in the literature are** and what areas need to be examined. Making yourself aware of relevant studies helps prevent duplicating what already has been done. Chapter 7; Evaluating the Evidence, will provide guidelines for conducting the literature review.

Another skill is learning how to identify good literature and research. This process also allows the researcher to discover what instruments or tools have been used to study the topic of interest, as well as the conceptual or theoretical frameworks applied. In the case of EBP, it also enables the researcher to determine if the evidence available advises a change in practice. Some questions may reveal a lack of evidence or research on a given topic. This should alert the researcher to the need for further research on the topic of interest.

Often, researchers ask how far back in the literature they should search. Generally, the researcher should look for relevant studies or literature within the past five years. However, if no research has been published within this time frame, the researcher will need to go back further. In either case, it is always appropriate to include landmark studies, even if they more than five years old. **Landmark studies** are studies that may be older than five years but are **paramount to the direction of study of the topic.**

Step Five: Identify a Theoretical or Conceptual Framework

Nursing research is not conducted just to learn the answer to a specific question or to test a hypothesis. When a study is placed in a theoretical context, it allows one to speculate on the questions of why and how treatments work and how variables relate to each other (Polit & Beck, 2004). **Theory provides the structure for a research study.** It allows the researcher to generalize beyond a specific situation and predict what should happen in similar situations (McEwen & Wills,

2002). Good research integrates findings into an orderly and coherent system. Meleis (2007) states that the goal of theory in research "is to formulate a minimum set of generalizations that allow one to explain a maximum number of observational relationships among the variables in a given field of inquiry" (p. 45). She further states that the relationship between theory and research is cyclical in nature. The result of research can be used to verify, modify, disprove, or support a theoretical proposition. Nursing theory has provided new propositions that would not have been articulated if theories from other disciplines were used. Nursing theory is, therefore, very important.

For example if a research study was conducted examining the level of comfort a patient experiences postoperatively without pain medications, the study could be guided by Katherine Kolcaba's comfort theory (2008) or Roy's adaptation model (Barone, Roy, & Frederickson, 2008).

The word theory can be used in many ways. Scientists use theory to mean "an abstract generalization that offers a systematic explanation of how phenomena are interrelated (Polit & Beck, 2004). It can also be categorized as descriptive, which Fawcett (1999) defines as an empirically driven theory that can be used to "describe or classify specific dimensions or characteristics of individuals, groups, situations, or events by summarizing commonalities found in discrete observations" (p. 15).

A **metaparadigm is a primary phenomenon** that is of interest to a particular discipline. (Fawcett, 2009). Within nursing, the primary or central phenomena are the concepts of person, environment, health, and nursing (Fain, 1999). Theories that deal with these four metaparadigm concepts are referred to as nursing theories.

There are also traditional nursing theories that differ in their level of generality. **Grand theories are complex and broad** in scope. They include many concepts that are not usually grounded in empirical data (i.e., data gathered through the senses using objective measurement) or evidence. Therefore, they are not very useful in creating guidelines for nursing practice (Fain, 2009). **Middle-range theories** are theories that **focus on only one piece of reality or the human experience, but involve a selected number of concepts** (e.g., theories of stress) (Polit & Beck, 2008). **Practice theories are more targeted than middle-range theories and produce specific directions or guidelines for practice.** An example is the Theories of End-of-Life Decision Making (Fain, 1999). **Prescriptive theories** are theories **that address nursing therapeutics and the outcomes of interventions.** A prescriptive theory includes propositions that call for change and predict the consequences of a certain strategy for nursing intervention (Meleis, 2007). **Borrowed theories are taken from another discipline,** for example psychology, and applied to nursing questions and research problems (Fain, 2009).

The building blocks of theories are called concepts. These are "words or phrases that convey a unique idea or mental image that is relevant to the theory" (Schmidt & Brown, 2009, p. 106). In other words, they describe a phenomenon, which is an aspect of reality that can be consciously observed, sensed, or experienced. Phenomena within a discipline such as nursing (for example, caring) reflect that domain (caring for a patient in nursing as compared to caring about what one will eat for dinner) (Meleis, 2007). As such, a concept gives some degree of classification or categorization (Meleis, 2007).

Constructs are higher level concepts that are derived from theories and represent non-observable behaviors (Fain, 2009). A conceptual model is the same as a conceptual framework, which is a set of abstract and general concepts assembled to address a phenomenon of central interest (Polit & Beck, 2008). It represents ideas or notions that have been assembled in a specific way to represent or describe a particular area of concern. Conceptual models are loosely constructed in comparison to theories (Fain, 1999).

So where does one find a nursing theory to use with a research study? See Table 3.6 for Web sites that provide information about nursing theories.

Step Six: Keep the Study Ethical

All studies should be conducted ethically. You must check if study participants were subjected to any physical harm, dis-

TABLE 3.6	Sources of Information on Nursing Theorists

Nursing theory Web page:
http://www.enursescribe.com/nurse_theorists.htm

Nursing theory page:
http://www.sandiego.edu/academics/nursing/theory/

Nursing theory network: http://www.nursingtheory.net/

comfort, or psychological distress. Did the researchers take appropriate steps to remove them from harm? Did the benefits to participants outweigh any potential risks? Did the benefits to society outweigh the costs to the participants? Was any type of coercion or undue influence used in recruiting or selecting the participants? Were vulnerable subjects used? Were the participants deceived or tricked in any way? Were they fully aware of participating in a study, and did they understand the purpose of the research? Were appropriate consent procedures used? Were appropriate steps taken to safeguard the privacy of participants? Was the research approved and monitored by an Institutional Review Board (IRB) or other similar ethics review committee? All of these things need to be considered when evaluating a research study.

Step Seven: Identify Study Assumptions

Assumptions are "statements and principles that are taken as truth, based on a person's values and beliefs" (Fain, 2009, p.192). **Assumptions are presumed to be true, but may not indeed have been proven.** Nieswiadomy (2008) describes three types of assumptions:

1. Universal assumptions. An example would be that all humans need love.
2. Assumptions based on a theory or research findings. For example, a study based on the finding that worrying leads to stress must identify the assumption that worry leads to stress so that a study on stress can use this assumption as its basis.

3. Assumptions that are necessary to complete the study. For example, if someone was studying women who commit murder and your study is conducted in a prison ward with convicted female murders, you can assume that the women indeed committed murder.

Every scientific study or investigation is based on assumptions. Therefore, the researcher should state these assumptions clearly so factors that may have influenced the questions asked and other parts of the study are identified.

Step Eight: Formulate the Hypothesis and/or Research Questions

The researcher's expected findings form his or her hypothesis. The **hypothesis** is what ultimately **predicts the relationship between two or more variables**. The problem statement asks the question of interest, and the hypothesis then predicts the answer. The hypothesis should contain the population of interest and the variables, just as the problem statement does. A hypothesis must be able to be tested in a real-life situation (Nieswiadomy, 2008). Remember that the independent variable is the "cause," and the dependent variable is the "effect." There are several types of hypothesis, but only a few will be discussed here.

A **research hypothesis** is a statement that shows an expected relationship among the variables. A **null hypothesis**, on the other hand, shows a complete lack of or absence or relationship among the variables (Polit & Beck, 2008). The null hypothesis is important when looking at statistics related to a study.

The **directional type** research hypothesis is preferred for nursing studies (Nieswiadomy, 2008). A directional hypothesis shows that a relationship exists among the variables, but that there is also an expected direction to that relationship. For example:

1. There is a relationship between increased smoking and the increased risk of acquiring lung cancer. (An obvious positive relationship is shown: increased smoking and increased risk of acquiring lung cancer.)
2. Older people are more susceptible to motor vehicle accidents because of slower reflexes than younger people. This predicts a relationship between increased accidents and aging, as reflexes are slowed or decrease. While this is an inverse relationship, it is indeed a directional relationship.)

A **nondirectional hypothesis** shows just the opposite; it shows that no direction exists among the variables. For example:

1. There is a relationship between diet and the risk of obesity. (*This does not clearly predict a direction, whereas the following statement would.*)
2. People who consume more than 3,000 calories per day will have an increased risk of being obese. (*This shows an increased caloric consumption and increase risk of being obese, and an obvious direction.*)

> ### Fast facts in a nutshell
>
> The purpose of research questions is to generate new knowledge, whereas the purpose of EBP questions is to make decisions about or that affect patient care

Research questions are statements that seek to address an identified research problem. In some cases, they are a direct rewording of the statement of purpose phrased as a question rather than a statement (Polit & Beck, 2008). For example, if the problem statement is to determine the difference between high carbohydrate diets and obesity, the purpose may be to examine the link between these elements. The research question(s) may be:

- Is there a correlation between diets of complex carbohydrates and increased obesity?
- Is there a decreased incidence of obesity among people who do not consume carbohydrates?
- Is there a family history that predisposes one to obesity?

Answers to the following can be used to develop research questions:

1. Is there a relationship?
2. What is the direction of the relationship?
3. What is the strength of the relationship?
4. What is the type of the relationship?

Step Nine: Identify the Type of Research Design

The most basic way of identifying the type of research design is to **ask if it is quantitative or qualitative.** Then, look at the factors for each type of study that will need to be addressed, including the population, how the data will be analyzed, and the communication of the results. These will be discussed in greater detail in Chapters 4 and 5.

Fast facts in a nutshell: summary

In summary, Florence Nightingale, while not an evidence-based researcher, is credited as the first nurse researcher because of her observations and notes made during the Crimean War. The two basic types of research are quantitative and qualitative. Each category includes multiple types of research. Basic steps in the research process are: 1) identify the problem to be examined (problem statement); 2) define the purpose of the study; 3) determine the study variables; 4) conduct a review of the literature; 5) identify a theoretical or conceptual framework; 6) keep the study ethical; 7) identify assumptions about the study; 8) formulate the hypothesis and/or research questions (what is it the researcher wants to know or predict); and 9) identify the type of research design you want to use. While these steps are not the only way to do research, they do provide a framework to guide you as you begin to understand the research process.

REFERENCES

Adams, S. (2009). Indentifying research questions. In N. A. Schmidt & J. M. Brown (Eds.), *Evidence-based practice for nurses: Appraisal and application of research* (pp 57–74). Boston: Jones & Bartlett.

Fain, J. A. (2009). *Reading, understanding, and applying nursing research* (3rd ed.). Philadelphia: F.A. Davis.

Fawcett, J. (1999). *The relationship between theory and research.* Philadelphia: F.A. Davis.

Gillis, A., & Jackson, W. (2002). *Research for nurses: Methods and interpretation.* Philadelphia: F.A. Davis

Houser, J. (2008). *Nursing research: Reading, using, and creating evidence.* Sudbury, MA: Jones & Bartlett.

LoBiondo-Wood, G., & Haber, J. (2006). *Nursing research: Methods and critical appraisal for evidence-based practice,* (6th ed.). St. Louis, MO: Mosby.

McEwen, M., & Wills, E. M. (2002) *Theoretical basis for nursing.* Philadelphia: Lippincott, Williams & Wilkins.

Meleis, A. I. (2007). *Theoretical nursing: Development and progress* (4th ed.). Philadelphia: Lippincott, Williams & Wilkins.

Nieswiadomy, R. M. (2008). *Foundations of nursing research* (5th ed). Upper Saddle River, NJ: Pearson.

*Nightingale, F. (1860). *Notes on nursing. What it is and what it is not.* New York: Appleton.

Polit, D. F., & Beck, C. T. (2010). *Essentials of nursing research: Appraising evidence for nursing practice* (7th ed.). Philadelphia: Wolters Kluwer/Lippincott, Williams & Wilkins.

Polit, D. F., & Beck, C. T. (2008). *Nursing research: Generating and assessing evidence for nursing practice.* Philadelphia: Lippincott, Williams & Wilkins.

*Considered a classic reference that helps define the discipline of nursing.

Chapter 4

Quantitative Research

INTRODUCTION

The two main research designs are quantitative and qualitative. This chapter discusses the basics of quantitative research designs. Chapter 5 discusses the basics of qualitative research designs.

Quantitative research has many designs, and the literature on the subject is vast. This chapter provides a brief overview of basic quantitative research designs, along with related key terminology needed to understand the basics of evidence-based practice (EBP). For further clarification of topics and concepts, consult a comprehensive and detailed nursing research textbook.

In this chapter, you will learn:

1. A basic overview of quantitative research.
2. The two basic designs of quantitative research: experimental and nonexperimental.
3. The "Hawthorne Effect."

4. Randomization.
5. How to complete a basic analysis of findings in quantitative research.

QUANTITATIVE RESEARCH

Quantitative research designs examine relationships between variables and are categorized as experimental or nonexperimental. In experimental designs, the researcher usually manipulates the experimental variables, there is a comparison group in the study, and the subjects are usually randomly assigned to the experimental or comparison group. The nonexperimental design is used when research cannot be conducted on human subjects because it would either be unethical or it would cause pain or harm to the subjects. Nonexperimental designs are descriptive and describe the phenomena as it exists. The researcher does not have control over the subjects and can only attempt to control for extraneous variables by carefully selecting the study sample. For a brief overview of experimental and nonexperimental designs, see Table 4.1.

DESIGNS IN QUANTITATIVE RESEARCH

Experimental Designs

True Experimental Design

In a true experimental design, the researcher has greater control over the situation because the rival or alternative hypoth-

TABLE 4.1   Quantitative Research Designs

Experimental designs	Nonexperimental designs
• True experimental design • Pretest-posttest control group • Posttest-only control group • Solomon four-group • Quasi-experimental designs • Nonequivalent control group • Factorial • Randomized block • Crossover/repeated measures • Time series • Preexperimental • One shot case study	• Descriptive studies • Action studies • Comparative studies • Correlational studies • Developmental studies • Evaluation studies • Meta-analysis studies • Methodological studies • Needs-assessment studies • Secondary analysis studies • Survey studies

esis can be ruled out as an explanation for the observed response (Fain, 1999). The three criteria necessary for a true experimental design are: 1) the researcher manipulates the experimental variables; 2) at least one experimental and one comparison group are included in the study; and 3) subjects are randomly assigned to either the experimental or comparison group.

The researcher also looks for a cause and effect (outcome). **All experimental studies involve the manipulation of the independent variable (cause) and, then, the measurement of the dependent variable (effect).** Several issues related to experimental design need to be mentioned. The first is that not all variables can be manipulated. For example, if you are studying patients who have pneumonia, the researcher cannot infect more patients with pneumonia so that they can be added to the study. That would not be ethical. So, when conducting an experimental research study or when reading a study to determine to what extent the researcher was able to control the variables involved, keep these points in mind.

Fast facts in a nutshell

All experimental studies involve the manipulation of the independent variable and, then, the measurement of the dependent variable.

Keeping a Study Ethical

Conducting an ethical study is very important. In the past, some studies were conducted without regard to human rights. The famous Tuskegee Syphilis Study is one such example. The study involved an experiment that lasted more than 40 years. It was designed to examine the long-term effects of syphilis in adult African American males, but many of the men studied were not aware that they were subjects. This violates the right of informed consent. In addition, when penicillin became available to treat syphilis, the government withheld the medication from this group so that the study could continue. Without the penicillin, many of the men died. Since that time, legislation has imposed important safeguards to prevent such an atrocity from happening again (Nieswiadomy, 2008). **Today, subjects in every study must give informed consent.** This means that *before* a researcher begins collecting data, he or she must make sure that each participant understands the nature of the research project and the implications of participating in the study. The researcher must provide information about the potential benefits and risks and ensure that the subject is participating voluntarily, without any coercion. Researchers also must also provide ample time for the subjects to ask questions and clarify any confusion about participation in the study. For children, a parent or custodian must give consent for the child to participate. "First do no harm," the most basic principle of medicine, applies to research as well as to the practice of medicine. In the research environment, it simply means that no subject shall be harmed during the process of data collection. This is extremely important. Consent to conduct a study must also be obtained from an institution's Internal Review Board (IRB). The IRB is a group of individuals who review and approve all studies before they are conducted. This ensures that human rights are protected and proper procedures or protocols are being followed so that no participant is harmed.

Fast facts in a nutshell

Subjects in every study must give informed consent.

For a **retrospective study**, one **looks back in time to data already obtained** and on record, regulations requiring informed consent do not apply, as long as the data does not identify the patient. However, the U.S. Health Insurance Portability and Accountability Act of 1996 (HIPPA) is very clear about the type of information that can be removed from patient records for the data to be considered de-indentified (Polit & Beck, 2008). HIPPA requires national standards for electronic medical information to keep health information private. An institution, such as a hospital, can disclose individually identifiable health information (IIHI) from its records if a patient signs an authorization allowing access. This authorization can be incorporated within a consent form or it can be a separate document (Polit & Beck, 2008). It is best to check with each institution as to its policies and procedures before looking at any patient data.

The **Hawthorne effect is an important phenomenon in experimental designs.** If a researcher is conducting a study and the subjects know they are indeed being studied, they may change their behavior, actions, or replies to questions during the study. That change of behavior is the Hawthorne effect. For example, suppose a nurse is conducting a study on the hand washing compliance of staff and is observing members of the staff walking in and out of patient rooms. The staff may become suspicious as to why the researcher is watching them. They may fear the researcher is monitoring their practices and, therefore, change their behavior and wash their hands more frequently than they normally would have done. This skews the results of the study. Waltz, Strickland, and Lenz (2005) note that subjects who are being observed usually notice the observer's presence and figure out they are being watched within approximately ten minutes.

Fast facts in a nutshell

The Hawthorne effect occurs when subjects change their behavior, actions, or responses to questions because they know they are being studied.

For a good experimental study to be conducted, there also needs to be randomization. **Randomization** is a procedure **that ensures that every subject has an equal chance of being chosen** for the experiment. There are numerous methods to achieve this goal. It can be done by computer-generated numbers, a random numbers chart, selection of every third person, or a simple flip of a coin. An experimental study usually has two separate groups of subjects: a true experimental group and a control group. When applying a variable, or intervention of interest, such as testing a new drug and its effects, the members of the experimental group would receive the drug and the members of the control group would not. The control group might also be referred to as the comparison group. To alleviate the Hawthorne effect, the researcher may choose to "blind" the study. **Blinding is when the subject does not know if they are in the experimental group or the control group.** For example, if the researcher is testing a new medication for depression, the subject will not know if he or she is getting the new medication or a placebo, which is a pretend, or fake, medication. A study can be single blinded or double blinded. Single blinding is one way. The subject does not know if they are in the experimental or control group. Double blinding is two way. It is when both the researcher and the subject don't know if the subject is in the experimental group or in the control group. In this example, neither the researcher nor the subject knows who is receiving the medication and who is receiving the placebo. **Double blinding is the most efficient way to eliminate any type of subjectivity or bias.** *Bias* is an important term that **means an influence of some sort on the study or outcome of the study.** This occurs when the researcher interjects his or her personal beliefs into the study, either knowingly or unknowingly. For example, assume a researcher is studying the positive effects of using sugar to sweeten coffee. First, the researcher is guilty of bias in the way the study is worded. It states a "positive" effect. How does the researcher know it will be positive? Secondly, the researcher may say to the subject, "Doesn't your coffee taste sweeter and better?" In this case, the researcher is planting ideas into the subject's head and altering the outcome of the experiment. That is a form of bias.

Fast facts in a nutshell

Double blinding is the most efficient way to eliminate any type of subjectivity or bias.

Quasiexperimental Design

In a **quasiexperimental design,** which is similar to an experimental design, **there is no randomization or comparison**

group. This type of study might be conducted when randomization is not possible. The researcher uses an already established group for the experimental group. This type of design is used with people in their naturally occurring groups, which is more like the "real world." For example, a researcher studying a group of Native Americans is working with a group that is predetermined by culture. This makes determining the cause-and-effect relationship weaker than in a true experimental design because the researcher is making generalizations about only one group of individuals, Native Americans. The researcher cannot assume that these findings would also be applicable to say African Americans. As a result, quasiexperimental designs are ranked lower on the hierarchy of rating evidence for EBP.

Nonexperimental Designs

A nonexperimental design is frequently used when experimental research cannot be conducted on human subjects. For example, if a researcher wants to study the effects of pain on children, it would be unethical to induce pain in asymptomatic children to conduct the study. The researcher cannot intentionally subject any one group to pain. All nonexperimental studies are therefore descriptive in nature. Because the researcher cannot manipulate or control variables, he or she can only describe the phenomena as they exist. The researcher can, however, try to control extraneous variables by carefully selecting the study sample. An extraneous variable is one that is not of interest to the researcher but can affect the study by causing an unanticipated effect. These can be called intervening, or confounding, variables. The two broad categories of nonexperimental design are descriptive and correlational. Survey studies, comparative studies, and methodological studies will also be discussed.

Fast facts in a nutshell

Nonexperimental designs include descriptive, correlational, survey, and methodological studies.

Descriptive Design Studies

Descriptive design studies describe in detail the phenomena of interest and the relationship among its variables. The purpose of descriptive designs is to observe and describe phenomena in real-life situations. In nursing, a descriptive design can be used to identify problems, make decisions, or determine what other people in similar situations are doing (Houser, 2008). For a descriptive study, information already exists in the literature about the phenomena of interest, while, for an exploratory study, no such information is available. An example of an **exploratory study** would be a researcher studying the use of a particular antibiotic, let's say antibiotic X. If antibiotic X is given intravenously, the researcher's question would be, "Does it cause venous irritation?" The researcher would describe what happens, if anything, when the antibiotic is given. The researcher is exploring a new situation and gathering new data and has no knowledge of a possible answer based on published reports. This is an exploratory study.

Remember that if the study is observational or descriptive in nature, the characteristics of the sample group are usually examined by methods such as questionnaires, surveys, interviews, and direct observation. Conclusions are made about the subjects or sample from these observations. The sample is usually divided, but may not be done randomly (Carlson, Kruse, & Rouse, 1999).

Correlational Design Studies

Correlational design studies are used to find relationships among two or more variables within a situation without knowing the reason for the relationship (Boswell & Cannon, 2007). In correlational studies, the researcher seeks to find the strength of the relationship between variables to see if a change in one variable results in a change in the other, that is, to see if there is a correlation between the two variables. The magnitude or direction of a correlation can be measured by using a positive or negative correlation coefficient. They range from -1.00 (a negative correlation) to 1.00 (a positive correlation). A correlation coefficient of $.00$ shows no relationship between the variables. Correlation coefficients can be reported through various statistics, such as Pearson's product moment correlation or Spearman's rho (Nieswiadomy, 2008). In reviewing evidence from a correlational study, remember that a correlation does not prove causality. In other words, just because a correlation was found between "A" and "B" does not mean that "A" caused "B." Correlational research simply seeks to find the "correlation."

Survey Studies

Survey studies obtain data through subjects' self-reporting about variables such as attitudes, perceptions, and behaviors. Surveys can be conducted face to face or over the telephone. The questionnaire is a popular method in collecting data (Peters, 2009). Survey tools are readily available, or the researcher may choose to develop his or her own. Remember that if the researcher develops a new survey tool, he or she must remember to test the new tool in a pilot study to confirm that it is valid and reliable. A **pilot study is a small-scale trial run** of a larger research project using a smaller number of subjects. In this case, the pilot study would be done to test the survey tool. Many of us have received surveys in the mail. **Cross-sectional surveys look at people at one point in time; longitudinal surveys follow subjects over a period of time.**

Some advantages of surveys are that the researcher can collect a large amount of information quickly at a minimal cost. Using survey tools, a researcher can reach large groups of a people in a shorter amount of time than is possible when conducting a face-to-face survey. Incentives may be offered for the participant to complete the survey. Short surveys are usually more effective than long and detailed surveys.

Comparative Studies

Comparative studies look at the difference between intact groups on some dependent variable of interest. While this sounds a lot like a true experimental study, the difference is in the extent to which the researcher can manipulate the independent variable. In comparative studies, there is no manipulation of the independent variable. For example, when looking at spousal abuse, it would not be ethical to examine abuse as an independent variable in one group and then choose another group whose members would not be abused.

Comparative studies frequently are classified as retrospective or prospective. In retrospective studies, the researcher looks backward in time. In prospective studies, the researcher looks for an effect in "real time" or in the future.

Methodological Studies

In methodological studies, nurse researchers look at "the method." This type of study is used most often to test instruments or analyze the development, testing, and evaluation of research instruments. For example, assume a researcher develops a tool to measure "happiness" in obstetric patients after delivery. The new "happiness scale" would need to be tested to see if it is indeed a valid method of measuring happiness. This would be done in a methodological study. Remember, the researcher is "testing the method."

A biophysiologic method tests an instrument of some kind. It is important that the biophysiologic instrument is calibrated to ensure accuracy, reliability, and validity before the study is started. An example of a biophysiologic method or an instrument is a glucose meter. If you are conducting a study about glucose levels using a new glucose meter, you would want to ensure that the meter is working properly before conducting the study.

> ## Fast facts in a nutshell
>
> It is important not to confuse exploratory and explanatory research.

Exploratory **research studies are conducted when little is known about the phenomena.** For example, a researcher might decide to determine the needs of the families of patients who go home with implanted vagal nerve stimulators. If a review of the literature demonstrates limited information on vagal nerve stimulators, it would be most appropriate to do an exploratory study.

In *explanatory* **research studies, the researcher searches for causal explanations or explanations of "why" or "how" phenomena are related.** This method is much more rigorous than exploratory or descriptive research. This is usually experimental type research. While in exploratory and descriptive studies, the researcher describes phenomena and examines relationships among phenomena, in explanatory research, the researcher provides an explanation for the relationships that are found among the phenomena (Nieswiadomy, 2008). For example, in the exploratory research on antibiotic X mentioned above, the researcher found out antibiotic X does cause venous irritation. In explanatory research, the researcher explains why the venous irritation happens. In this case, it could be related to the pH of antibiotic X.

ANALYSIS OF FINDINGS IN QUANTITATIVE RESEARCH

The analysis of data, along with both descriptive and inferential statistics, can be mind boggling for the person new to research and goes beyond the scope of this book. For more detail on this type of data analysis, consult a basic research text. However, a brief explanation of the following three simple principles—level of significance, confidence intervals, effect size, and standard deviation—will be discussed. See Table 4.2 for a basic guide for critiquing quantitative research.

TABLE 4.2   Guide to Critiquing Quantitative Research

Critiquing Guidelines

What type of quantitative study was done?
- Does the process relate to the type of study?
- Does it make sense?

Is the design of the study identified and does it fit the hypothesis or answer the research questions?
- What designed was used?
- Does it make sense for this type of study?
- Will this type of study test the hypothesis presented?

What were the results of the study?
- What are the results?
- How were they obtained and measured statistically?
- Is this significant?
- Will the results help locally or impact clinical practice?

(continued)

Critiquing Guidelines *continued*

Is the measurement reliable?
- Does it measure the same thing on repeated measures?
- Is the study re-producible?

Are the results valid?
- Does the study measure what it is supposed to?
- Is there any bias present?
- Are there any confounding variables?

More Specific Questions

What is the measurement effect?
- What is the number of participants in the study? (n= _____)
- Are the two groups (control & experimental) evenly divided?

Are the results of the study clinically significant?
- If they are significant at what level?

How was the sample size decided?
- Was there any randomization?
- Was there any blinding of the subjects?

How was the data analyzed?
- What statistical tests were used if any?
- Was there a significant p value?

Level of Significance

The level of statistical significance is written as a "**p value**." A "p value" measures how much evidence we have against **the null hypothesis** (which is how much of a chance we have in saying the null hypothesis is wrong). In nursing, for a result to be considered significant, it must have a "p value" of less than 0.05. **If the p-value is less than 0.05, the result is significant. If the p value is greater than 0.05, the result is not considered significant.**

More simply, if a report indicates that the findings are significant at the 0.05 level, that means that only 5 times out of 100 (5 divided by 100 or 0.05) would the obtained results be incorrect. In other words, 95 out of 100 times, the same results (a positive correlation or relationship) could be obtained with another sample or test. This is the same as saying that a null hypothesis (no correlation or relationship between variables) will be rejected only 5 times. You can have a high degree of confidence that these results are reliable. So a p-value of less than 0.05 is good. A p-value of less then 0.01 is better. Look at the p-values in Table 4.3. Which is less than 0.05?

Keep in mind that while the "p" value tells you that a difference exists between the experimental and control group, it does not tell you the magnitude of the effect. To understand the magnitude of the effect, you would need to understand the clinical and statistical significance, which involves looking at confidence intervals and effect size (Rempher & Silkman, 2007).

Confidence Interval

Confidence intervals are computed on the mean and standard deviation. If a study has a confidence interval of more than 95%, that is good. This means that the data is correct 95% of the time. So a 99% confidence interval is better than a 90% confidence interval.

Confidence intervals reflect the degree of risk researchers are willing to take of being wrong. With a 95% confidence interval, the researcher accepts the probability that they will be wrong only 5 times out of 100 (Polit & Beck, 2008).

Effect Size

An effect size is the magnitude of the relationship between two variables, or the magnitude or difference between two groups with regard to some attribute of interest (Polit & Beck, 2008). Although an intervention or variable is expected to have an impact on the outcome and be reported as clinically significant, this may not translate into actually being clinically significant (Houser, 2008). For example, suppose a researcher is studying the effect of aerobic exercise on heart rate and losing weight. While the relationship is strong, an effect will be seen with a small sample size. However, if it was found that exercise had little effect on the heart rates of patients with hyperthyroidism, a much larger sample would be needed to find any significant changes in heart rate in this study. So where you have a strong relationship among variables, a small sample might be possible to show that relationship. But, where the strength of the relationship among variables is not as strong, or where another intervening variable might affect the results, a much larger sample of subjects will be needed.

Standard Deviation

A standard deviation shows the average amount that values deviate from the mean. The mean is simply the average of a set of numbers. For example, if you add 10, 11, and 12, you come up with 33. If you then divide that sum (33) by the total numbers in the example (3), your mean, or average, is 11. A standard deviation is a useful variability index for describing a distribution and interpreting individual scores in relation to other scores in the sample. Similar to the mean, the standard deviation is a stable estimate of a parameter and is the preferred way of determining a distribution's variability. This is only appropriate for variables measured on an interval or ratio scale.

For a standard deviation you want a result as close to the number 1 as possible. It can be positive or negative. So an SD of +0.9 is good. An SD of +3.0 is worse. An SD of −1.0 is good, but an SD of −5.7 is bad. The absolute measure is zero, so the closer you get to zero the better. See Table 4.3 for an example of p-values and standard deviation.

TABLE 4.3	Example of p-Values and Confidence Intervals	
Interview #	Standard deviation	p-value
Interview #1 ($n = 35$)	1.33	.014
Interview #2 ($n = 40$)	1.05	.057
Interview #3 ($n = 50$)	0.91	.008 (significant)
Interview #4 ($n = 34$)	1.00 (good)	.011

Fast facts in a nutshell: summary

1. The two main types of research are quantitative and qualitative. Quantitative research is further divided into experimental and nonexperimental.
2. A variable is something that can be measured, like blood pressure and heart rate. The independent variable influences the dependent variable. The independent variable is the "cause," and the dependent variable is the "effect."
3. Randomization is a way that subjects are chosen for a study. With randomization, every subject or participant has an equal chance of being selected.
4. Bias occurs when researchers interject their feelings or personal beliefs into the study in a way that might affect the outcome of the study.
5. Retrospective studies look backward in time, and prospective studies look at issues in "real-time" or in the future.

REFERENCES

Boswell, C., & Cannon, S. (2007). *Introduction to nursing research: incorporating evidence-based practice.* Sudbury, MA: Jones & Bartlett.

Carlton, D. S., Kruse, L. K., & Rouse, C. L. (1999). The research column: Critiquing nursing research. A user friendly guide for the staff nurse. *Journal of Emergency Nursing, 25*(4), 330–332.

Fain, J. A. (1999). *Reading, understanding, and applying nursing research* (2nd ed.). Philadelphia: F.A. Davis.

Houser, J. (2008). *Nursing research: reading, understanding, and creating evidence.* Sudbury, MA: Jones & Bartlett.

Polit, D. F., & Beck, C. T. (2008). *Nursing research: generating and assessing evidence for nursing practice* (8th ed). Philadelphia: Lippincott, Williams & Wilkins.

Nieswiadomy, R. M. (2008). *Foundations of nursing research* (5th ed). Upper Saddle River, NJ: Pearson.

Peters, R. M. (2009). Quantitative designs: Using numbers to provide evidence. In N. A. Schmidt & J. M. Brown (Eds.), *Evidence-based practice for nurses: Appraisal and application of research* (pp 57–74). Boston: Jones & Bartlett.

Rempher, K .J., & Silkman, C. (2007). How to appraise quantitative research articles. *American Nurse Today, 2*(1), 26–28.

Waltz, C. F., Strickland, O. L., & Lenz, E. R. (2005). *Measurement in nursing research* (3rd ed.). New York: Springer.

Chapter 5

Qualitative Research

INTRODUCTION

The second main type of research is qualitative research. Qualitative research is more subjective and is based more on life experiences than quantitative research, which involves datasets of numbers. It involves smaller groups of subjects, often includes narratives, and attempts to identify common themes. The researcher collects data until saturation is achieved. This chapter explores the characteristics of four types of qualitative research: phenomenological, ethnological, grounded theory, and historical. Case studies, narratives, feminist research, and community-based participatory action research (PAR research) are other types of qualitative research.

In this chapter, you will learn:

1. A basic understanding of qualitative research.
2. How to examine the process of knowing.

3. How to explore the basic types of qualitative research, which include:
   • Phenomenology.
   • Ethnography.
   • Grounded theory.
   • Historical research.
4. How to examine other examples of qualitative studies, including case studies, community-based participatory action research, feminist research, and narrative research.

WHAT IS QUALITATIVE RESEARCH?

Qualitative research is not easily defined. It requires the examination of the quality of something rather than its quantifiable elements. It infers a subjective interpretation. LoBiondo-Wood and Haber (2006) believe that qualitative research is about human experiences. It frequently is conducted in natural settings and uses words or text rather than numerical data to describe the experiences being studied.

Before the 1970s, qualitative methods were used primarily in anthropology and sociology. Then, during the 1970s and 1980s, qualitative research methods were adopted by researchers in education, social work, management, nursing, and women's studies (Tilley, 2007). **Qualitative research lends itself effectively to the nursing process, which focuses on the person as a whole.** Over the years, its methods have become valued in the science of nursing, as the nursing process looks at the continuum of care from assessment to diagnosis to planning to interventions to an evaluation of care given.

Clearly, not everything a nurse experiences can be reduced to numbers and physiological measurement. The experienced nurse knows that there is more—more to nursing that is sometimes left unsaid and unexplained.

Fast facts in a nutshell

Qualitative research requires the examination of the quality of something rather than its quantifiable elements. It lends itself effectively to the nursing process, which focuses on the body, mind, and spirit of the individual.

THE PROCESS OF KNOWING

How does a nurse "know" or sense when a patient is going to crash or deteriorate? How does a patient "get the feeling" that he or she is going to die? Sometimes, nurses just know, but how does one get to this place of knowing. Is it through learning or acquiring facts? Is it instinctive? Or, is it something more? Most importantly, how can it be measured in the research process?

Have you cared for a patient and just "sensed" something was wrong? How did you know? Was it a feeling, a sometimes overwhelming feeling? What if you work in the Emergency Department (ED) or in the Intensive Care Unit (ICU)? Have you experienced the feeling that your patient was "going to crash" or was "about to die?" How and why did you get that feeling? How did you know? How can you measure that?

Michael Polanyi

Michael Polanyi, a professor of physical chemistry and social science, made significant contributions to the fields of philosophy and social science. He referred to this type of knowing as "tacit knowledge." He believed that creative acts (especially acts of discovery) are shot through, or charged with, strong personal feelings and commitments (personal knowledge). Polanyi said that these personal hunches, informed guesses, and imaginings are part of exploratory acts that are motivated by what he called passions. He felt these "hunches," or this prelogical phase, occurred because we "knew more than we could tell" (Infed, 2003). It is an interesting concept to explore. More information about Polanyi can be found on the Web at http://www.missouriwestern.edu/orgs/polanyi/.

Patterns of Knowing

Barbara Carpers' (1978) patterns of knowing try to explain how we know what we know. Carper discusses four types of knowing: empirical, personal, ethical, and aesthetic. Empirical knowledge is what we know through our physical senses. This is something we can hear, touch, taste, and see. These are best handled through quantitative methods of discovery. Ethical knowledge requires that we make moment-to-moment decisions about what is right, what should be done, and what is good? This knowledge directs our personal conduct. Personal knowledge concerns the inner experience we have. It is the shared human experience and humanistic qualities of knowing. Aesthetic knowledge is abstract and gives us an appreciation of the deeper meaning of the situation. It takes an inductive approach to knowledge acquisition. These four patterns of knowing make it evident that the nurse who wants to research aesthetic knowing, in particular, will find a qualitative method more appropriate than a quantitative method.

Fast facts in a nutshell

Barbara Capers' four types of knowledge are empirical, ethical, personal, and aesthetic.

TYPES OF QUALITATIVE RESEARCH

Although many types of qualitative research can be conducted, only the four main types will be discussed here. Remember, in qualitative research, the people who are being studied are called "participants" or informants" rather than "subjects," which is the term more frequently used in quantitative research.

For researchers who are beginning to plan a qualitative study, it is important to consider exactly what you as the nurse researcher are interested in studying or exploring. Table 5.1 presents a decision path that provides guidance in choosing the correct type of qualitative research to use. Remember, for an evidence-based project (EBP), you will not conduct an actual research study, but rather gather "evidence" to examine your topic of interest.

Qualitative research does not begin with a hypothesis. The researcher does not begin such a study by predicting the

TABLE 5.1 Qualitative Decision Path

If you are interested in:		Method to consider is:		A question to ask might be:
Understanding the personal and human experience	⇒	Phenomenology	⇒	What is the "lived" experience?
Uncovering a social experience	⇒	Grounded Theory	⇒	How does this social group react to. . . ?
Learning about how a culture responds, feels, and reacts	⇒	Ethnography	⇒	How does this cultural group view or perceive caring?
Understanding the past through collection, organization, and critical appraisal of the facts	⇒	Historical Research	⇒	What caused an outbreak of polio in the past that may contribute to the outbreaks of today?
Obtaining unique stories and examples	⇒	Case Study	⇒	How do Native Americans value health care?
Exploring the gender domination and discrimination within patriarchal societies	⇒	Feminist Research	⇒	How do women make decisions?

results. To avoid bias, the researcher should be free of pre-conceived notions (bracketing) and be de-centered, so he or she can become immersed in the situation. In the qualitative study, the researcher becomes the "research tool," or the research instrument. To accomplish this, a researcher must clear his or her mind and put personal thinking aside. Otherwise, bias may become part of the study.

One way that a qualitative researcher gathers information is through interviews. While conducting an interview, the researcher may take field notes by using a recording device or taking notes to ensure accurate recall of statements, thoughts, and information gathered. An interview may contain too much information for the researcher to trust to memory. These notes may be written during the interview session if not too distracting for the participant, or may be written after the interview is completed. Sometimes during the interview, unusual mannerisms may be present. It may be important for the researcher to include these mannerisms in their field notes. For example, if during an entire interview, the informant is wringing his or her hands and sweating profusely, the researcher should record this in a field note since this might signify nervousness or tenseness.

Fast facts in a nutshell

- In the qualitative study, the researcher becomes the "research tool," or the research instrument.
- A researcher must clear his or her mind and put personal thinking aside.
- Field notes about an interview help the researcher remember the essential facts.

Phenomenology

Phenomenology is a qualitative approach that explores the meaning of the human condition through the "lived experience" of the individual. The researcher mainly uses dialogue to explore each participant's history. Phenomenology describes the meaning that experiences hold for each participant. It examines the "humanness" in life. It is important to mention that the participants or informants are asked to describe their experiences as they perceive them. The researcher must separate his or her feelings and not impose them on the research participants. This process is known as bracketing. *Bracketing* is the process that requires researchers to identify their own personal biases about the phenomenon of interest and to clarify how their personal experiences and beliefs may alter what is heard and reported (LoBiondo-Wood & Haber, 2006). The research question may sound something like this: "What is the lived experience of women in abusive relationships?"

Fast facts in a nutshell

- Phenomenology explores the experiences of the individual.
- Bracketing is the process that requires researchers to identify personal biases and not impose them on the research participants.

Writing the Open-Ended Question

The research question guides the entire study, so it must be worded correctly, focused, and open ended. The question asks about human experiences in a given situation. This question is not exactly the same as the first question or any question used to initiate the dialogue with the participant. For example, while the research question may be, "What is the lived experience of women in abusive relationships?" the statement or question that will initiate the dialogue with the participant could be, "Tell me what it is like to live with your husband?" or "What is your relationship like?" It is important not to impose bias into an opening question. Therefore, an inappropriate question would be, "Tell me what it is like to live in an abusive relationship?" This particular question assumes and makes a judgment that the relationship is abusive. While the relationship may be abusive, it is not the researcher's place to tell or suggest to the participant that the relationship is abusive.

Purposive Sampling

Where does one get the sample for a phenomenological study? The researcher will need to engage in purposive sampling. In this type of sampling, the researcher uses his or her own judgment in selecting people who will be representative of the group the researcher is interested in exploring. For example, the researcher may go to a battered woman's shelter to study the lived experiences of women in abusive relationships. The researcher would not want to go to a church recreation social or a marriage encounter weekend getaway, where the chance of finding participants who are abused might be low. The researcher wants to go to a place where the population of interest would be found. Sometimes the researcher may need a key informant. **A key informant is a person who is knowledgeable about the population of interest**; they are also used in ethnographic studies. The informant might also be able to provide the researcher access to the designated population. This may be the director of the woman's shelter, who has known the women for quite some time. If the director introduces the researcher to the women, the women may open up more readily to the researcher. The researcher should spend time at the place of interest, in this case a woman's shelter, so that the participants or informants get to know and learn to trust the researcher. This is called **immersion**. The researcher must become immersed in the population of interest to fully gain insight and understanding into what it is like to experience the lived experience being studied. It is hard to understand anything if, for example, you don't know the language. So, it is important for the researcher to become fully immersed in the population of interest to understand that population.

Fast facts in a nutshell

To select an appropriate sample:
- Go to a place where the population of interest will be found.
- Find a key informant, a person who is knowledgeable about the population of interest.
- Immerse yourself in the population of interest.

Mode of Data Collection

Data may be collected in a number of ways. **In-depth interviews are usually the primary way phenomenological data is obtained.** These interviews may be audiotaped or videotaped depending on the informants comfort level. This data acquired must then be transcribed by the researcher or, because the work is tedious, by a hired transcriptionist. Once the data is transcribed, similar or common themes are identified. The researcher can accomplish this through the use of note cards or notes or through use of a computer program designed to make this part of data collection and analysis easier. Examples of this type of programs are *NVivo, Nudist,* or *Atlas/t.* The researcher continues to collect data until a point of saturation is reached. **Saturation** is when common themes are found, and no new information is obtained. For example, the researcher exploring abused women interviews six informants, who all tell the researcher the same thing, such as, their significant others often drink alcohol before abusing them. Then, it is safe for the researcher to say that drinking was a common theme of precipitating abuse in women. If this saturation of data has occurred, the researcher can stop the interview process. This is why fewer informants may be needed in a qualitative study. The researcher keeps interviewing informants until saturation is obtained. Saturation could occur after 5 interviews or after 12 or more interviews.

Ethnography

Ethnography, ethnographic studies, or ethnonursing studies are qualitative studies that explore the cultural aspects of a particular group of informants. According to Germain, (2001), ethnography is the "systematic description, analysis, and interpretations of cultures or subcultural groups" (p. 277). In the United States, ethnography emerged in the early twentieth century in the field of cultural anthropology. Margaret Mead is one of the well known proponents of this type of work (Germain, 2001). **Ethnography seeks to understand the values, norms, customs, rules, and ways of life that categorize the group of interest.** This understanding may take place through the use of interviews, observations, reading documents, examining photographs, videotapes, looking at genograms, or a combination of these approaches. **A genogram is a pictorial diagram of a person's family relationships and medical history.**

Before starting an ethnographic study, bracketing is essential to free yourself of predetermined prejudices or biases. In ethnographic research, immersion is both vital and necessary. The best way for the researcher to understand the culture is to live in the culture. Again, the use of a key informant who assists the researcher in gaining access to the particular group of interest is helpful. It is important to note that a culture does not have to represent a nationality. **A culture can be any group of individuals with similar beliefs, behaviors, rituals, or patterns of life.** For example, a group of mothers who are primary caretakers of children with chronic illnesses can be considered a culture. Nurses can be considered a culture. Also, a culture can contain subcultures. For example, within the culture of the medical profession, nurses, physicians, and nursing assistants or aids can each be considered a subculture.

Ethnographic researchers explore phenomena within a culture from the "emic" perspective. **Emic means intrinsic,** or from the internal perspective. For example, a researcher exploring the emic perspective of Native Americans is doing so from the perspective of the Native American. This means that the resulting study would reflect the point of view of Native Americans in giving reasons for their beliefs and customs.

If the researcher were exploring phenomena from an "etic" perspective, the researcher would be examining the life of the Native American from an extrinsic or external perspective. This means that the resulting study would represent the researcher's interpretation of the same Native American custom or belief. The etic perspective usually takes on a more analytical perspective.

In ethnographic studies, it is important to do fieldwork or live with the informants in their natural environment. This environment could be people's homes, tribal areas, reservations, huts, or any areas the informant considers home or a place of existing.

Madeline Leininger has done extensive work in developing her "Sunrise Model," which grew out of her Culture Care Theory. This theory was developed in the 1950s and 1960s. Her 1991 book, *Culture Care Diversity and Universality,* offered a breakthrough concept in exploring the nursing care given to individuals who were culturally different from the nurse caregiver. Her work continued with the development of the theory of transcultural nursing, in which Leininger (2002) states the purpose was to discover and explain cultural-based factors that influence the health, well-being, illness, or death of individuals of a cultural group. Leininger (1978) also proposed ethnonursing, which is essentially a new method for nurse researchers that includes "the study and analysis of the local or indigenous people's viewpoints, beliefs, and practices about nursing care phenomena and processes of designated cultures (p. 15). Leininger defines ethnography as "the systematic process of observing, describing, documenting, and analyzing the life ways or particular patterns of culture (or subculture) to grasp the life ways or patterns of the people in their familiar environment, (p. 35). Ethnography and ethnonursing remain valued areas of interest for many nurse researchers.

Fast facts in a nutshell

Madeline Leininger applies ethnographic research methods to nursing. She proposed the term *ethnonursing* to describe the study of the nursing practices and beliefs among indigenous people.

Grounded Theory

Grounded theory is a qualitative approach developed by two sociologists, Glaser and Strauss (1967). The researcher studies, collects, and analyzes data before developing a theory grounded in that data (Richards & Morse, 2007). Researchers use grounded theory when they are interested in describing social processes from the perspectives of human interactions or "patterns of action and interaction between and among various types of social units" (Denzin & Lincoln, 1998). The goal of grounded theory research is to understand how a group of people defines their reality through social interactions. It uses an inductive (i.e., from the ground up) approach using everyday behaviors or organizational patterns to generate a theoretical explanation (Munhall, 2001). In this type of study, the researcher uses purposive sampling to look for informants who can shed light on the topic being explored. The emergent theory is based on observations and perceptions of the social scene and evolves during data collection and analysis as a product of the actual research process (Strauss and Corbin, 1994). Data collection is continued until saturation has occurred.

Fast facts in a nutshell

Grounded theory is an inductive approach to research that uses purposive sampling for finding informants who can shed light on the topic of interest.

Historical Research Method

The historical research method is a based on documentation of sources that retrospectively examine events or people (Schmidt & Brown, 2009). This method gains understanding of the past through the collection, organization, and critical appraisal of the facts. One of the main goals of this type of research is to shed light or a new interpretation on past events. When critiquing this type of study, be aware that the research question may be implied rather than clearly stated. A second important point about historical research is that the more clearly the researcher identifies the historical event being studied, the easier it will be to identify more specific data sources. In examining the sources of data, it is important to determine if the data come from primary or secondary sources. **Primary data sources** include eyewitness accounts of the time being studied that is an account by someone who was actually present (LoBiondo-Wood & Haber, 2006). Other examples of primary sources would be oral histories, written records, diaries, eyewitnesses, government documents, pictures, or physical evidence related to the time specified. **Secondary sources** provide a view or recounting of the event that is not a first-hand, eyewitness account (LoBiondo-Wood & Haber, 2006). This could be an account of an event interpreted using primary sources as the basis for that interpretation.

> ### Fast facts in a nutshell
>
> The historical research method uses data from primary sources (contemporary records and accounts) or secondary sources (subsequent interpretations of events based on primary sources).

OTHER TYPES OF QUALITATIVE STUDIES

Case Studies

Case studies involve the study of an issue through one or more cases within a bounded system or setting (Creswell, 2007). A case study can examine institutions and facilities, such as an in-patient psychiatric unit. Cases studies review the peculiarities and commonalities of a specific case, which is familiar ground for practicing nurses. A case study is not a methodological choice, but rather a choice of what to study. It can include quantitative and or qualitative data, but it is defined by its focus on an individual case (Stake, 2000). The two types of case studies are intrinsic and instrumental. An **intrinsic case study** is used to develop a better understanding of the case—it is nothing more or less. The researcher sorts out other curiosities, so that the stories of "those living the case" will be teased out (Stake, 2000). For example, assume a researcher examines incarcerated mothers. In an intrinsic case study, the researcher would interview two women who previously participated in a study about drug usage and were now in jail. The researcher would ask them about their lives after being arrested and jailed. This provides an insight into the women's experiences. Both women regretted using drugs and being incarcerated. It could be concluded that these data could guide practice and future research about this issue.

An **instrumental case study** selects one case study to illustrate an issue of concern (Cresswell, 2007). An example would be a researcher who would like to challenge the notion that all patients diagnosed with Down Syndrome are mentally challenged and of lower intelligence than the general population. The researcher would look at a case in which a person with Down Syndrome is not only is holding a job, but is the manager at a local restaurant chain. With this evidence in an instrumental case study, the data obtained could be used to change not only perceptions, but prejudices, and to guide further research.

Community-Based Participatory Action Research

Community-based participatory action research requires that the community actively participate in all stages of the research process (LoBiondo-Wood & Haber, 2006). After identifying a problem, the researcher, together with the community, explores possible solutions, the method of studying the problem, and the analysis of the data obtained. This is an excellent method for solving community-based problems. It proposes that if the community is involved in the process, members may be more apt to "own the project," participate in the project, implement the project, and bring the project to a completion or outcome. An example is research on the increase in violence in the community related to gangs and drugs. The community comes together with the researcher to determine a plan to address the situation, implement the plan, evaluate the plan, and, in the process, solve or eliminate the problem. If the problem has not been solved or eliminated, perhaps information was uncovered that could be used to further assess and develop new possible solutions.

Feminist Research

This type of research approach focuses on gender domination and discrimination within patriarchal societies. The researcher seeks to establish a nonexploitive relationship with his or her informants and to conduct research that transforms these perceived boundaries (Polit & Beck, 2008). An example of feminist research would be the decision making of postpartum women in choosing whether to breast feed their babies. Is discrimination involved in their decision-making process? Feminist research seeks to uncover and define these real or perceived boundaries of gender.

Narrative Research or Storytelling

One type of research approach that is gaining popularity is narratives, or storytelling. This type of research allows people to "tell their stories" so that their motivations, desires, and feelings in a multitude of settings are uncovered. Narrative research has many forms, uses a variety of analytic processes, and is rooted in the social and humanities disciplines (Daiute & Lightfoot, 2004). Polit & Beck (2008) believe that narrative analysis focuses on the story as the object of inquiry to see how individuals make sense of their lives and environments.

SUMMARY

Qualitative approaches to research inquiry are a viable way to explore or examine situations or problems that are not easily measured by quantifiable methods. Qualitative research is growing in popularity and use by the nursing profession in trying to explain more humanistic situations in which the "lived experience" of individuals may be influenced by variables not identified through quantitative research. The qualitative approaches mentioned in this chapter, along with others, give nurse researchers the ability to study those aspects of life and nursing care that are not easily quantifiable, but require abstract thought or in-depth examination of how the individual human relates to or fits in the overall picture of health care. For questions to ask in critiquing a qualitative study, see Table 5.2.

TABLE 5.2 Guide to Critiquing Qualitative Research

Critiquing Guidelines	YES	NO
Ask yourself:		
What were the results of the study?		
• Is the phenomenon or topic of interest clearly identified?	❏	❏
• Does the research approach fit with the purpose or aim of the study?	❏	❏
• Are the conclusions of the study consistent with the results are reported in the study? (No jumps or reaches for conclusions.)	❏	❏
Are the results valid?		
• Were the study participants chosen appropriately?	❏	❏
• Is that consistent with the type of study conducted?	❏	❏
• Was accuracy and completeness of the study guaranteed?	❏	❏
• Do the findings fit the data from which they were generated?	❏	❏
Will the results help me take better care of my patients?		
• Are the findings relevant to people in similar situations?	❏	❏
• Did the reader learn any new important information?	❏	❏
• Does the research relate to or change practice?	❏	❏

More Specific Questions	YES	NO
Did the researcher indicate the type of study approach?		
• Are the language and concepts consistent with the study approach?	❏	❏

(continued)

- Are the data collection and data analysis consistent with the study approach?   ❏   ❏

Is the significance/importance of the study clear?
- Does the review of the literature support the need for a study?   ❏   ❏
- Does the study make a difference to current practice?   ❏   ❏
- Are the background and significance of the study defined?   ❏   ❏
- Are the implications for future research specified?   ❏   ❏

Is the sampling method clear and appropriate for the type of study?
- Does the researcher indicate the sample size and demographics?   ❏   ❏
- Does the researcher control the selection of the sample?   ❏   ❏
- Is the type of sample appropriate for the type of study?   ❏   ❏
- Is the number of sample participants appropriate for the type of study?   ❏   ❏

Is the way the data was collected clear?
- Are the sources and methods of verifying data clear?   ❏   ❏
- Are the researcher's roles and actual involvement clearly explained?   ❏   ❏

Adapted from Melnyk & Fineout-Overholt (2005).

Fast facts in a nutshell: summary

1. The four patterns of knowing articulated by Carper are empirical knowledge, ethical knowledge, personal knowledge, and aesthetic knowledge.
2. The four main types of qualitative research are phenomenology, ethnography, grounded theory, and historical research. Other types include case stud-

ies, narratives or story-telling, feminist research, and community-based participatory action research, among others.

3. Remember that in qualitative research, the people in the study are called participants. In quantitative research, they are called subjects.

4. Saturation is when you reach a point in a qualitative study where all the participants are giving you the same responses. You have reached a point of saturation at which no new data will be forthcoming.

5. Madeline Leininger (1991) developed "The Sunrise Model," in which transcultural nursing seeks to discover and explain cultural-based factors that influence health, well-being, illness, or death of individuals of a cultural group.

6. The difference between primary and secondary sources is that primary sources include eyewitness accounts to the event being examined, while secondary sources are written by people who heard or read about the event or occurrence via a primary source. Primary sources are much more desirable for accurate accounts of basic information.

REFERENCES

*Carper, B. (1978). Fundamental patterns of knowing in nursing. *Advances in Nursing Science, 1*(1), 13–23.

*Considered a classic reference that helps explain the process or theory.

Cresswell, J. W. (2007). *Qualitative inquiry and research design: Choosing among five approaches.* Thousand Oaks, CA: Sage

Daiute, C., & Lightfoot, C. (2004). *Narrative analysis: Studying the development of individuals in society.* Thousand Oaks, CA: Sage.

Denzin, N. K., & Lincoln, Y. S. (1998). The art and politics of interpretation. In N.K. Denzin & Y.S. Lincoln (Eds.), *Handbook of qualitative research* (2nd ed.). Thousand Oaks, CA: Sage.

Germain, C. P. (2001). Ethnography. In P. L. Munhall (Ed.), *Nursing research: A qualitative perspective* (pp. 277–306). Boston: Jones & Bartlett.

Glaser, B., G., & Strauss, A. C. (1967). *The discovery of grounded theory: Strategies for qualitative research.* New York: Aldine.

Infed. (2003). *Michael Polanyi and Tacit Knowledge.* Retrieved July 22, 2007 from http://www.infed.org/thinkers/polanyi.htm

*Leininger, M. (2002). Culture care theory: A major contribution to advance transcultural nursing knowledge and practice. *Journal of Transcultural Nursing, 13*(3), 189–192.

*Leininger, M. (1998). Ethnography and ethnonursing: Models and modes of qualitative data analysis. In M. Leininger (Ed.), *Qualitative research methods in nursing.* Fort Worth, TX: Harcourt College Publishers.

*Leininger, M. (1991). *Culture care diversity and universality.* Sudbury, Massachusetts: Jones & Bartlett.

Leininger, M. (1978). Caring: The essence and central focus of nursing. *The phenomenon of caring.* American Nurses Foundation Nursing Research Report, Part V, 1977.

LoBiondo-Wood, G., & Haber, J. (2006). *Nursing research: Methods and critical appraisal for evidence-based practice* (6th ed.). St. Louis: Mosby.

Munhall, P. L. (2001). *Nursing research: A qualitative perspective* (3rd ed.). Sudbury, MA: Jones & Bartlett.

Nieswiadomy, R. M. (2008). *Foundations of nursing research* (5th ed). Upper Saddle River, NJ: Pearson.

Polit, D. F., & Beck, C. T. (2008). *Nursing research: Generating and assessing evidence for nursing practice* (8th ed.). Philadelphia: Lippincott, Williams, & Wilkins.

Richards, L., & Morse, J. M. (2007). *Users guide to qualitative methods.* Thousand Oaks, CA: Sage

Schmidt, N. A., & Brown, J. M. (2009). *Evidence-based practice for nurses: Appraisal and application of research.* Sudbury, MA: Jones & Bartlett.

Stake, R. (2000). Case studies. In N. Denzin & Y. Lincoln (Eds.), *Handbook of qualitative research* (pp. 435–454). Thousand Oaks, CA: Sage

*Strauss, A., & Corbin, J. (1994). Grounded theory methodology. In N.K. Denzin & Y.S. Lincoln (Eds.) *Handbook of qualitative research,* Thousand Oaks, CA: Sage.

Tilley, D.S. (2007) Qualitative Research Methods. In C. Boswell & S. Cannon (Eds.), *Introduction to nursing research: Incorporating evidence-based practice.* Sudbury, MA: Jones & Bartlett.

Chapter 6

Finding the Evidence

INTRODUCTION

The two basic formats for articles you will use for your research evidence are print and electronic. Print sources remain available at most libraries, but much information is now available electronically and is therefore readily accessible to anyone with access to the Internet.

In this chapter, you will learn:

1. The difference between primary and secondary sources.
2. How to explore print and electronic sources.
3. The basic databases and search engines available when searching for evidence.
4. How to conduct a basic literature search.

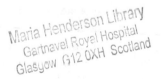

PRIMARY VERSES SECONDARY SOURCES

In research in any field, a primary source is one written by the person(s) who conducted the research study or wrote about the topic of interest. Secondary sources are a description of a study or article written by someone else. It is preferable when searching for evidence to use only primary sources.

PRINT SOURCES

How does one begin to research an evidence-based practice project? The **print sources can be found in the library using indexes**, which contain references to articles in periodicals that have been published over a period of years. These print indexes can be used to locate journal articles related to the topic of interest.

Cumulative Index to Nursing and Allied Health Literature (CINAHL)

The *Cumulative Index to Nursing and Allied Health Literature* (CINAHL) has been published continuously since 1961. Until 1977, the title was the Cumulative Index to Nursing Literature. CINAHL now includes nursing and allied health journals, including dental hygiene, nutrition, occupational therapy, physical therapy, physician's assistant, and respiratory therapy journals. This print index is a bound text found in the periodical section of the library. Do not hesitate to ask the librarian for assistance. Most libraries have research assistants available to help novice researchers. CINAHL is also available online in a electronic database that now is owned and operated by EBSCO Publishing. Information about CINAHL is available at http://www.ebscohost.com/cinahl/. A subscription to this database is required, so it is easiest to access through an educational institution or workplace that maintains a subscription. Sometimes, you are able to print full-text articles. In other cases, you will only be able to obtain a reference and an abstract of the article. This varies depending on the type of subscription purchased. Most often references and abstracts are free to the general public without a subscription.

Nursing Studies Index (NSI)

The *Nursing Studies Index* was compiled at the Yale University School of Nursing under the direction of Virginia Henderson. This index is an annotated guide to English language reports of studies and historical and bibliographical materials about nursing. The four available volumes, published from 1963 to 1972, cover the years 1900 to 1959. This is an important resource for studies conducted during the first 60 years of the 20th century.

Index Medicus

This is the best-known index of medical literature. First published in 1879, the last printed volume appeared in December 2004. Since 1977, this database is available for free on the Internet through MEDLINE.

Abstracts

An abstract is a brief summary of an article's contents that describes its purpose, methods, and major findings. By reading an abstract, the researcher should be able to understand the highlights of the article and determine if it is related to the topic of interest. The abstract, which is usually the first paragraph underneath the title, is identifiable by its appearance; it is usually indented or printed in boldfaced of italic type.

The abstract described above is the basic one you will find with a research article. Other styles of abstracts that you may discover during your search include psychological abstracts, dissertation abstracts, and masters thesis abstracts.

Fast facts in a nutshell

A database is a collection of data or information stored in a computer system. Think of it as an electronic filing system.

ELECTRONIC SOURCES

Electronic sources have become the preferred method of accessing research articles and literature. The use of electronic communication has changed both the way data is searched and obtained. The world of electronic databases can be accessed most often through one's home computer. Many schools, universities, and medical institutions also provide access to electronic databases.

Databases

The key to finding data or articles pertinent to your study is to access the appropriate database. There are many to choose from. Some are free, and some must be purchased by universities or medical institutions. For example, MEDLINE can be accessed free through the National Library of Medicine's PubMed search system. A full bibliographic source is given. Some are free, but some publishers may charge a fee to purchase a full-text article. See Table 6.1 for examples of common searchable databases and additional information.

Bibliographic Sources

A bibliographic source, whether printed or on the Web, simply provides you with a complete reference that you can use to locate the full-text article.

Abstracts

An abstract is simply a concise summary of a research article that is designed to help the reader quickly grasp the key elements of the article. The abstract usually includes the research problem or issue addressed, the type of research method used, the results or findings of the study, and the main conclusions or recommendations from the study. Some databases on the Web provide free abstracts. Others require you to purchase that information. See Table 6.1 for more information on such.

TABLE 6.1 Examples of Databases	
Database	Description
CINAHL (Cumulative Index of Nursing and Allied Health Literature) (1982–present) • Material from more than 3,000 journals. • Full-text is available for more than 300 journals, but must be purchased. • Abstracts and bibliographic references are also available. • It is owned & operated by EBSCO publishing. • More information is available at http://www.ebscohost.com/cinahl/	Premier site for nursing and allied health. Also includes nutrition, physical therapy, occupational therapy, dentistry, and respiratory therapy journals
EBSCO host, an international information system that provides e-journals, e-book, and print subscriptions, as well as e-resource and management tools, full-text and secondary databases, and related services • Has more than 300 full-text or secondary databases available. • Includes bibliographical citations, abstracts, full-text articles, and provides other references where the article is cited	Provides clinical patient-oriented, administrative databases with the latest bedside evidence, nursing resources, education materials, marketing tools, medical research databases, social work information, and the ability for CME and CEU opportunities

(continued)

Database	Description
• Multilanguage health databases available • Free trials are available, but must be purchased • More information and a downloadable brochure is available at http://www.ebscohost.com/uploads/thisTopic-dbTopic-1015.pdf	
OVID is operated by the Wolters Kluwer Health publishing company. Internationally supported. • Includes full bibliographical references, abstracts, full-text links, authors full name reference, other articles citing the article found. A paid subscription is needed to use this database. • Search aids are suggested on the screen • Education support and tutorials are available free of charge. • Available in multiple languages	Key subject areas include agricultural and food sciences, bioengineering and biotechnology, clinical medicine, computer science and technology, dentistry, earth, and environmental sciences, evidence based medicine, geology and life sciences, neurology and neurosciences, nursing and allied health, pharmacy, philosophy and religion, physics, psychology and psychiatry, social sciences and the humanities, technical science, veterinary medicine, and zoology.
PubMED was developed by the National Center for Biotechnology Information (NCBI) at the National Library of Medicine	Includes primarily general science and chemistry journals, for which the life sciences articles are indexed for MEDLINE.

(continued)

Database	Description

(NLM), located at the U.S. National Institutes of Health (NIH).
- Publishers participating in PubMed electronically submit their citations to NCBI prior to or at the time of publication. If the publisher has a Web site that offers full-text of its journals, PubMed provides links to that site as well as biological resources, consumer health information, research tools, and more. However, there may be a charge to access the text or information.

MEDLINE (Medical Literature Analysis and Retrieval System Online) (1966-present)
- Includes article full citation.
- Provides links to many (but not all) full-text articles and other related resources
- The largest component of PubMed
- A free accessible online database of biomedical journal citations and abstracts created by the U.S. National Library of Medicine (NLM®). Approximately 5,200 journals published in the United

Studies in medicine, nursing, dentistry, psychiatry, veterinary medicine, and pharmacy.

(*continued*)

Database	Description

States and more than 80 other countries have been selected and are currently indexed for MEDLINE.
* Available from the NLM home-page and can be searched for free at http://www.nlm.nih.gov

ERIC (Education Resources Information Center Institute of Education Sciences) (1966-present). An index of education journals • Contains more than 1.3 million bibliographic records of journal articles, the majority are peer reviewed • Abstracts and links to full text in PDF format are available from individuals and publishers who give free full text. Web sites and libraries that may have full text are provided. For most materials from 2004 forward, if full text is not available in ERIC, links to publishers are provided. • Contains journal articles, books, research synthesis, conference papers, technical reports, policy papers, and other education-related materials.	Studies from the world of education. ERIC indexes materials from scholarly organizations, professional associations, research centers, policy organizations, university presses, the U.S. Department of Education, and other federal, state, and local agencies. Individual contributors submit conferences, papers, research papers, dissertations, and theses.

(continued)

Database	Description
PsycINFO (corresponds to the print *Psychological Abstracts*) (1887-present) • This is an abstract database • Prepared by the American Psychological Association. • Contains more than 2 million records selected from more than 2,000 journals • Also contains bibliographic citations, abstracts, cited references, and descriptive information to help you find what you need across a wide variety of scholarly publications in the behavioral and social sciences.http://www.apa.org/psycinfo/	Studies from psychology and related disciplines. Usually accessed through a vendor like OVID or APA.
Cochrane Database of Systematic Reviews Excellent source for "evidence" in evidence based practice. • This includes full text of reviews • Abstracts of review are available at http://www.cochrane.org	Full text of systematic reviews prepared by the Cochrane Collaboration. Completed reviews and protocols.

Full-Text Databases

When searching for research articles look for sources that offer the "full text" of each article, including graphs, charts, and other illustrations. Vendors, such as OVID, include hyperlinks to references of full-text articles. The full-text article may be available in .pdf or .html format.

Fast facts in a nutshell

A hyperlink lets you click on a Web address that automatically connects (or links) you to relevant material. Hyperlinks usually appear in bold type, underlined, or in a different color from the rest of the text.

Key Word Search

Most electronic databases require that you begin a search by identifying key words. Key words are terms that describe your subject of interest. For example, when searching for information about incarcerated women with human immunodeficiency virus (HIV), use the key words "incarcerated women," "HIV in prison," "HIV in prisoners," "prisoners with HIV," or "AIDS in women." Trying each of these key words will demonstrate how the manipulation of a few words can yield different lists of research articles.

Search Engines

A **search engine is an information retrieval system stored on a computer system,** such as the World Wide Web. One of the most popular engines is Google, which was started in 1998.

Other search engines include:

- Dogpile.com
- Excite
- Yahoo search
- MSN search
- Ask.com (formerly Askjeeves.com)

The key to finding scholarly research articles is to use a search engine that yields reliable information. One free source that fits this requirement is Google Scholar, which can be used to locate nursing research articles. It also indexes other resources that are not part of scholarly studies, such as:

- Commercial sites.
- Individual home pages..
- Advocacy sites.
- Cheaters' sites.

Remember that unlike scientific and scholarly literature and databases, Google is unfiltered, so the user should be very careful. See Table 6.2 for the pros and cons of using Google scholar (http://www.googlescholar.com).

If you choose to use Google Scholar, you will find the following sources:

- Journal articles and abstracts
   * Publishers' Web sites (e.g., JSTOR, Muse, Wiley)

- * Free online databases (e.g., PubMed, ERIC)
- * Online journal sites (both free and subscription based)
- Peer reviewed papers
- Selected books from
  - * Google book search
  - * Open WorldCat

One important point to remember is that students are using Google scholar, which provides free access. Nurse scholars and other researchers are now citing it. Occasionally, Google scholar covers nursing literature better than traditional databases. So, indeed, use it as a search engine if you want to be comprehensive, but use it in addition to CINAHL, Medline, and other more traditional health information search engines. It may be helpful for topics that cross disciplinary boundaries. Google scholar is not currently a comprehensive source for serious research, but it continues to grow and improve (See Table 6.2).

TABLE 6.2   Pros and Cons of Google Scholar

Pros	Cons
• Cross disciplinary	• Lacks advanced search features
• Subjects don't neatly fit into one category	• No stated editorial policy
	• No controlled vocabulary
• Includes both book and journal literature	• Lacks standards for names
• Cited reference searching	• Coverage is inconsistent
• Citation checking	• Reports state that indexing labs PubMed by months

CONDUCTING A BASIC LITERATURE SEARCH

Starting the Search

Now that you have accessed a database, how do you conduct the actual search? It is important to understand some terms that will assist in the search. To start a search on "pediatric burn care," for example, access the computer's search engine and key in "burns" in the search box as your **key word**, the word you choose for your search that describes your topic of interest.

Fast facts in a nutshell

Remember that certain diseases can be known by different terms, so you need to search on all of them to get a complete list of the relevant literature.

Example: SUBJECT HEADING: CEREBRAL VASCULAR ACCIDENT
Can also be known as:
• stroke
• CVA
• cerebrovascular accident
• cerebral vascular accidents
• cerebrovascular accidents
• CVAs
• stroke

The CINAHL database will be used in this instructional example. You can access this database on your computer at http://www.ebscohost.com/cinahl/ and follow along with the search below.

The Initial Search

After typing in the term "burns" into the search window, the resulting search yielded 8,170 journal articles. It is clear by this large number of articles that this search term was too broad. The next step is to refine the search by combining two key words from your topic of interest: pediatrics and burns. By inserting the word "**AND**" as your **operator** between the key terms, the two terms will be connected, and the search will be more clearly defined. So, enter the refined search "burns AND pediatrics" and then hit search. This search will now deliver articles that contain both the terms "burns" and "pediatrics." The results have now identified 91 journal articles related to "burns and pediatrics."

Narrowing the Search

Narrowing the search by using two key words produced results that more exactly apply to the topic in which you are interested. The search has narrowed the results to 91 articles that relate specifically to pediatric burns.

To narrow the search even further, put "quotation marks" around the words used as your key terms. Doing this will yield only titles that contain both your key search words. See below about "using quotation marks when searching" or add more key words to refine your search even further.

Note that conducting a search using key word(s) is only one search approach. Searches also can be conducted using author name, article title, or journal title. In addition, searches can be basic searches, advanced searches, or searches that look for a specific citation in the text of an article. Simply select the method you want to use in conducting the search.

It is preferable to obtain articles that have "full text," so that you will be able to read them. To determine which articles are available as "full-text" articles, either:

1. scroll through all the articles to look for "full-text" articles, or
2. when conducting the search, click "linked full text" in the "limit your results" box on the right side of the screen.

Narrowing the search using a timeline is also possible. Note that the box on the side of the screen includes a timeline that shows the years for which the journal articles are available. To refine the search to reflect certain years, click "update results."

After updating, the search results lists only seven articles that have full text. These full-text articles are available as .pdf files, .html files, or linked files. Click on the desired text format to obtain the full text of the selected journal article. Also note that the timeline has also narrowed to the years 1999 to 2007 from the broader timeline previously displayed.

Expanding the Search

If, unlike the above example, the search using a key word only produced one hit, or result, the search would need to be expanded. To expand a search, enter the key word and then use the term OR and Truncation to increase your results. **Truncation is a term used to find variant word endings** as illustrated in the examples that follow:

Key Term	=	Truncations
Child*	=	child, children, children
Parent*	=	parent, parents, parenting
Spouse*	=	spouse, spouses, spousal

The truncation symbol varies by search engine. For example:

Search Engine	Truncation symbol to use
EBSCO host (CINAHL), Proquest, & Others	*
Ovid and Medline	$
Google, Yahoo	automatic

To expand your search using the CINAHL database truncation symbol, key in burns*. This will expand the search to include any articles that contain the word "burns" anywhere in the citation. Note that using the search term burns* could produce articles written by an author named Burns, articles that include burns in the title of the article, or articles that simply mention the term burns once in the text.

Be aware that different key words can generate dramatically different results. For example, if the word "children" was substituted for the word "pediatrics,"the search yields only two results, and they are not even full-text articles. Do not become frustrated when this occurs. Conducting a search takes time. Be creative, "free think," and search using a variety of terms to experience how different search results can be.

Use of Other Terms to Expand or Narrow Your Search

Boolean Search Operators

Boolean logic defines logical relationships between terms in a search. The Boolean search operators are **and, or,** and **not.** Please note that when executing a search, "and" takes precedence over "or."

- *And* combines search terms so that the text of each search result contains all of the terms. For example, **burns and pediatrics** finds articles that contain *both* burns and pediatrics
- *Or* combines search terms so that each search result contains at least one of the terms. For example, **burn or pediatrics** finds results that contain *either* burn or pediatrics.
- *Not* excludes terms so that each search result does not contain any of the terms that follow it. For example, **television not cable** finds results that contain television but *not* cable (EBSCO help, 2009).

Explode

To expand the subject heading, click explode. The headings are exploded to retrieve all references indexed to that term as well as all references indexed to any narrower subject terms. In this example, only "burns, inhalation" can be exploded. To explode these terms, check the box "explode" and click on smoke inhalation. In a database with a "tree," such as *MeSH* or *CINAHL*, exploding retrieves all documents containing any of the subject terms below the term you selected. In other databases, exploding retrieves all documents containing the selected term, as well as any of its first level of narrower terms. If a plus sign (+) appears next to a narrower or related term, there are narrower terms below it. Scan the list for a relevant term and click in its checkbox. Then click continue. This will then find articles related to those subheadings.

Major Concept

If you want to search by major subject heading, select "Major Concept." This creates a search that finds only records for which the subject heading is a major point of the article. Searches are limited with specific qualifiers (subheadings) to improve the precision of the search. Major subject headings indicate the main concept of an article. Note that you can **use both explode and major concept at the same time** to retrieve references indexed to your term (and its narrower terms) and all articles for which the subject heading is the major point of the article (EBSCO help, 2009).

Scope Notes

In some databases (e.g., *CINAHL, MEDLINE*), you can click on the word "scope" or the scope icon. This enables you to view the entire scope note, which is a explanation of a term and its synonyms.

> ### Fast facts in a nutshell
>
> To focus your search on specific terms, try putting "quotation marks" around the word(s).

Using "Quotation Marks" When Searching

When searching a database or using a search engine, **use quotation marks to enclose the search terms for your search**, such as "adult day care." If quotation marks are not placed around the search terms or phrase, the results will include references that contain any of the three words. Narrowing the search to the exact terms in this way will make the search more successful in producing articles that reflect the topic of your research.

For example, enter the search term "adult day cares." The following article will appear. Note that the citation contains all three words.

1. *Adult day cares and public policy: a strategic plan for the Louisville metropolitan area.* Wishnia GS; Kentucky Nurse, 1997 Oct-Dec; 45 (4): 5

If you enter adult day cares without quotation marks, your search will yield articles with just one of the words in them, as seen in the following three listings.

1. *Causation and intent: persistent conundrums in end-of-life care.* Rich BA; Cambridge Quarterly of Healthcare Ethics, 2007 Winter; 16 (1): 63–73

2. *Fostering the transition from pediatric to adult neurosurgical care.* Abraham S; AXON/ L'AXONE, 2007 Winter; 28 (2): 13

3. *What kills one woman every minute of every day?* Kantrowitz B; Newsweek, 2007 Jul 2–9; 150 (2): 56, 57

Searching by Publication or Journal

If the search produces a reference or citation to a journal article that you would like to use, locate the journal in a database by searching for the name of the publication or journal. To do this, click on the publication tab and search alphabetically by the first letter of the name of the journal to see if the database has your journal.

COMMON DATABASES

EBSCO host™

EBSCOhost can help you quickly find the articles needed to get your research papers and other assignments done in record time. EBSCOhost puts all the e-journals available at your library in a single place on the Web, so you don't have to jump all over the place to find the articles you need. With EBSCO-host, you can:

- **Find a specific journal** quickly by using the Find Journals feature.
- **Browse through a list of all journals** available with the Browse feature.
- Browse a list of **subject categories**, then view a list of all journals that fall in a category of interest. This allows you to easily find journals that cover specific topics.
- **Find specific articles** quickly using the Find Articles feature. Search by article title or by the author's name.
- **Find articles that cover a specific topic** by searching for key words in the titles, abstracts, and even full text of millions of articles.
- Read article abstracts and **link directly to full text** of the articles you find.

A citation you may find in EBSCOhost is:

Hepatitis A seroprevalence and risk factors among day-care educators. **(includes abstract)** Muecke CJ; Clinical & Investigative Medicine, 2004 Oct; 27 (5): 259–64 **(journal article - research, tables/charts)** PMID: 15559862 CINAHL AN: 2005114261
PDF Full Text HTML Full Text Linked Full Text

You can then just click on PDF Full Text and receive the full text article in a PDF format. Or, you can opt to receive the full text article in an HTML file. Also note that clicking on the linked full-text tab will hyperlink you to a site where you can access full text or may automatically download the full text format for you.

OVID Online

Ovid is another database you can use to conduct a search. Ovid Technologies is an international leader in electronic medical, scientific, and academic research information solutions. It is an operating company of Wolters Kluwer Health, a leading provider of information for professionals and students in medicine, nursing, allied health, pharmacy and the pharmaceutical industry. Ovid consists of hundreds of databases, including more than 1200 journals and books from dozens of publishers. Ovid offers training programs to assist you with your search. This and more information about Ovid can be found on line at http://www.ovid.com/site/help/training.jsp?top=28&mid=33 (Wolters-Kluwer Health, 2009). Another on-line tutorial for OVID(c)2008 is available at http://calder.med.miami.edu/pointis/ovidsearch.html

An Example Using the OVID Database

When beginning any search, you need to think of a search term. In the example below, "geriatrics" is your search term. As such, it would yield the following, which indicates 5,456 results:

Results of your search: geriatrics.mp. [mp=title, abstract, full text, caption text]
Viewing 1–10 of 5456 Results

That is a lot of articles to search through. Below, listed as number 14, is one example of the search you might see, with its reference information. Somewhere in this article "geriatrics" is mentioned. You see this is quite broad and may not be what you are looking for specifically.

14. U.S. Preventive Services Task Force * Screening for Chlamydial Infection: U.S. Preventive Services Task Force Recommendation Statement. Annals of Internal Medicine. 147(2):128–134, July 17, 2007.

So, you might want to refine your search by adding another search term. Perhaps "geriatrics and stroke" might yield more specific results. To the right of the citation on the OVID screen is a list of options. Click on the one that best fulfills your needs. If you only want the reference, click on that and it will give you the specific information you want.

- Complete Reference
- Table of Content
- Ovid Full Text
- Full Text
- Abstract

<u>Complete Reference</u> will give you just that—a complete reference of the article.

<u>Table of Contents</u> will give you the contents of a book or periodical.

<u>Ovid Full Text</u> will give you the full text with the journal name at the top of the article.

<u>Full Text</u> will give you the full text of the article with the database name on the top of it.

PUBMED

PubMed Central (PMC) is the U.S. National Institutes of Health (NIH) free digital archive of biomedical and life sciences journal literature. PubMed is a service of the U.S. National Library of Medicine that includes more than 17 million citations from MEDLINE and other life science and biomedical journal articles back to the 1950s. PubMed includes links to full text articles and other related resources. All the articles in PMC are free (sometimes on a delayed basis), as is access to available abstracts. To access more information about PubMed please visit its Web site at http://www.pubmedcentral.nih.gov/

Journals and Magazines

When you are looking for journal articles, be sure that you use only research articles published in scholarly journals. In contrast, magazines and some journal articles may not be written by a researcher or even by an expert in the field or a member of the medical profession. In such cases, you are actually reading someone else's opinion about the research; this is sometimes presented in an editorial format.

Therefore, it is important to look at both the author and the source of the information you are using. You would want to read research articles written by the researcher or an expert in your area of interest. It is most important to pay attention to the type of journal or magazine. The field of nursing has many nursing journals—and they are not called magazines. These journals can be online or in paper format. For many specialties, such as pediatrics, you will find many relevant journals whose articles are written by physicians, nurses, scientists, editors, and other professionals. Look at the journal to see if it offers research findings or just informational articles about a particular disease process or clinical application. While these may be very important, they do not lead to compelling evidence in EBP. If you recall the hierarchy of strong evidence, research from randomized controlled trials is the strongest evidence. You will not find that in journals that offer information-type articles. So you will need to look to a scholarly journal that includes only peer-reviewed articles. Please see below for more information about this type of journal.

Online Journals

A large number of journals are now available on-line. These journals may be referred to as **e-journals** or **e-zines.** At http://www.nursingcenter.com, you can view the contents of the most current issue of 50 journals. You can also go directly to each journal's home Web page, where you can usually view the most current issue of the journal. For example, if you are looking for a pediatric journal you can enter "pediatric nursing journals" into any search engine, such as Google, and a multitude of journals will pop up. If you are interested in geriatric journals, you can do enter "geriatrics" and geriatric journal sites will appear. See Table 6.3 below for a sample listing of nursing journals on-line that are free to access.

TABLE 6.3   Free Online Nursing Journals

Journal	URL
• All nurses.com (Web journal about critical care and emergency nursing)	www.allnurses.com
• *Imprint* (magazine for nursing students) from the National Student Nurses Association (SNA)	www.nsna.org
• *Internet Journal of Advanced Nursing Practice* (peer reviewed journal)	http://www.ispub.com/ostia/index.php?xmlFilePath= journals/ijanp/front.xml
• *Journal of Undergraduate Nursing Scholarship* (also provide links to other free scientific medical journals	http://www.ispub.com/ostia/index.php?xmlFilePath= journals.xml
• *Nursing World*	www.nursingworld.org/onj
• Online Journal of Issues in Nursing	www.nursingcenter.com/home
• Online Journal of Nursing Informatics	http://www.eaa-knowledge.com/ojni/

Scholarly Journals and Peer-Reviewed Journals or Articles

Scholarly Journals

A scholarly journal contains articles written by scholars, researchers, professors, or experts in the field on topics related to that journal. The journal has a review process in place and less emphasis is placed on advertising. It usually includes research articles that are of interest to other professionals in that field.

Peer-Reviewed Articles

If an article is peer reviewed, it means that it has been read and approved for publication by experts in the field of the research topic. Usually, more than one reviewer's approval is required for publication. The review process is usually blinded, which means that the reviewers do not know the name of the author so that personal relationships do not enter the process. All identifying author criteria and credentials are omitted from the article prior to the review process. (See Table 6.4 for the differences between magazines and scholarly journals).

Table 6.5 lists a sampling scholarly journals that you might want to consult in your search for research journals appropriate to your topic of interest.

TABLE 6.4 Differences Between Magazines and Scholarly Journals

	Magazines	Scholarly Journals
Author	Journalist; layperson; sometimes unknown. May be scholar, but not necessarily in the field covered.	Identified expert, scholar, or professor in the field.
Notes	Few or no references or notes	Includes notes and/or bibliography.
Style	Journalistic; written for average reader	Written for experts; shows research.
Editing	Reviewed by one or more persons employed by the magazine	Editorial board of outside scholars reviews articles before accepted for publication.
Audience	General public	Scholars or researchers in the field.
ADS	Many, often in color	Few or none; if any, usually look for books and other "scholarly" items.
Look	Glossy, many pictures often in color	More sedate look, mostly print.
Frequency	Usually weekly or monthly	Usually quarterly or monthly.
Contents	Current events; general interest	More specialized; research topics.
Indexes	Found in general periodical indexes (e.g. Readers Guide)	Found in subject specialized indexes.

The above table adapted from http://lib.mnsu.edu/research/documents/scholarly.pdf. Please visit this Web site for more information about scholarly journals.

TABLE 6.5	Scholarly Nursing Journals for Research

Advances in Nursing Science Journal
Canadian Journal of Nursing Research
Clinical Nursing Research
Dimensions of Critical Care Nursing
Evidenced Based Nursing
Journal of Advanced Nursing
Journal of Nursing Research
Journal of Nursing Scholarship
Nursing Research
Nursing Science Quarterly
Western Journal of Nursing Research

Fast facts in a nutshell: summary

Now that you have found a research article, how do you know it is a good one? Remember the principles you learned in the quantitative and qualitative chapters. Make sure the articles are relevant and follow the sound principles of research. Evaluate the evidence. We will explore this in the next chapter.

REFERENCES

Cumulative Index to Nursing & Allied Health Literature (CINAHL) database. (2009). Available online at http://www.ebscohost.com/cinahl/

Cochrane Collaboration of Systematic Reviews. Available online at http://www.cochrane.org/reviews/clibintro.htm

EBSCO help (2009). Thesaurus. Retrieved May 21, 2009 from http://support.ebsco.com

Henderson, V. (1978). *Nursing studies index* (6th ed.), Vols I-IV. New York: Macmillan

Nieswiadomy, R. M. (2008). *Foundations of nursing research* (5th ed.). Upper Saddle River, NJ: Pearson.

OVID Technologies (2009). Available online at http://www.ovid.com/site/index.jsp

PubMed. (2009). Available online at http://www.ncbi.nlm.nih.gov/pubmed/

PsycINFO (2009). Available online at http://www.apa.org/psycinfo/

Wolters Kluwer Health. (2009) *Ovid.* Retrieved June 15, 2009 from http://www.ovid.com/site/index.jsp?top=1

Chapter 7

Evaluating the Evidence

INTRODUCTION

Now that you have found your research article how do you know if it is a good research article or if it is a flawed one? When doing an evidence-based practice project, it is very important that you use reliable evidence. You would not want to recommend a change to a clinical practice based on evidence that is not "good" or on the basis of one study. This chapter discusses how to evaluate the evidence that you have found in order to design your EBP proposal.

In this chapter, you will learn:

1. To evaluate the evidence you found asking 4 key questions
2. Critique research articles using a simple worksheet
3. Understand the rating hierarchy of the evidence

EVALUATING THE EVIDENCE

Now that you have found evidence, you need to determine if the evidence is good enough to warrant a recommendation to suggest a change in practice. It is essential that the evidence be carefully scrutinized. You would not want to propose a change in practice based on flawed or biased information.

To determine if a study is relevant to your evidence-based practice project, you will need practice in analyzing the research. You may want to consult a research text for a more detailed understanding of this process. In this chapter, we will briefly discuss how to analyze evidence. Remember that just because a research study is published in a peer-reviewed journal does not ensure that it was well designed or well conducted. It does not guarantee that the data was accurately analyzed or that it was accurately reported in the publication. You need to think about how the study was designed, how the research was carried out, and how the data was analyzed. If a tool was used in the study, was it tested prior to use and proven both reliable and valid? Some general questions you may want to ask when examining studies are listed in Table 7.1. Also review Tables 4.2 and 5.3, which offer guides to critiquing quantitative and qualitative research.

> ### Fast facts in a nutshell
>
> Never suggest or recommend changing practice on the basis of one study. Many novices who embark on an evidence-based project (EBP) are so happy to find one study on the topic that they base their entire project on this study. This should never be done.

TABLE 7.1	Some Basic Questions to Ask When Evaluating Research Evidence

- Is the research study relevant or important to nursing?
- Is the abstract present, and does it include the purpose, method, and summary of findings of the study?
- Was there a theoretical or philosophical framework used for the study?
- Is there a hypothesis?
- How many subjects/participants are there?
- Is the number of subjects/participants relevant for the type of study done?
- How were the subjects selected?
- What method of data collection was used?
- Was the data collection method sound and accurate?
- Did the data collection method provide reliable and valid results?
- How was the data analyzed, and was it appropriate for the study?
- Are there any assumptions given for the study?
- Are there limitations given for the study?
- Are there suggestions for future research?
- Is there a discussion of the results?
- Is there any bias revealed in the data?
- Is there any researcher bias? For example, was the study done using students from a college where the researcher works? Does the study recommend a medication when funds to conduct the research were provided by the manufacturer of the medication?
- Were any ethical situations discussed, or were any ethical procedures violated?
- Was IRB approval and informed consent obtained prior to the start of the study?

As you begin to evaluate or analyze the evidence for your EBP, you need to ask yourself four key questions about the results of the study?

1) Are the results valid?
2) Are the results reliable?
3) Will these results help me provide improved care for my patients?
4) Do these results make sense for my patient population?

Lets take a look at each of these questions more closely.

1. What were the results of the study?

What exactly are the results of the study? Do they make sense and answer the research question(s)? For example, in a quantitative interventional study, how significant are the treatment effects? Is there a significant difference between the patients who received the intervention and those who did not? If not, then the study does not prove the intervention is successful, and no practice change should be recommended based on these results. In a qualitative study, did the research approach fit the purpose of the study? Was it congruent? In other words, did the results of the study make sense and answer the research questions? The results should be a logical explanation of the intent of the research project and should not be erroneous or answer a question other than the research questions. For example, if you are looking at the effect of a nursing intervention in the lived experience of parents of children with a chronic illness, what common threads or themes were found? Do they make sense? Do they fit in the context of the situation or living environment? Did the nursing intervention make a difference or not? If it did not, there would be no need to employ that intervention in your practice. If it did make a difference and the caregiver is telling you that it did, examine this intervention further to determine if it might work with your patient population or in your situation.

2. Are the results valid?
Validity means that the results measure what they were supposed to measure. For example, in an experimental or interventional study, were the participants or subjects randomly assigned to control, treatment, or intervention groups? Were they equal on key characteristics prior to the study? Were intervening or extraneous variables controlled? For example, your research study is measuring whether taking acetaminophen (Tylenol) every four hours around the clock keeps a child from getting a fever. Did the results show the child was fever free or did the child get a fever? If the results showed the child got a fever, then the purpose of the research study (to take acetaminophen every four hours around the clock) did not prove the hypothesis. Thus, you would not want to develop a protocol stating that administering acetaminophen every four hours around the clock will eliminate a child's fever.

3. Are the results reliable?
Does the research study measure what it is supposed to measure on subsequent experiences? Take the previous example with acetaminophen. If the research did report that giving acetaminophen every four hours alleviated fever, did this happen just one time or did it happen consistently for all subjects in the research study? In addition, if one research study shows that giving acetaminophen every four hours around the clock alleviates fever and another study shows that it does not, the second study negates the findings of the first study, and the

study results are not conclusive. So based on these two research studies, a practice change should not be implemented.

4. Will the results help me provide improved care for my patients?

Were the subjects or participants in the study similar to the patients of interest in your study? Are the benefits of the intervention or treatment greater than the inherent risks? Will implementation of these results make a difference in caring for my patients? Let's say that you are working with adult patients. Can you say that the results of the pediatric study with acetaminophen can be applied to adult patients? No, you cannot. If you are a pediatric nurse, will the results of these two studies help you in caring for children? No, because the two studies contradict each other. Are the benefits of giving acetaminophen every four hours (the intervention) greater than the inherent risk? Let's say that you give acetaminophen every four hours around the clock for several days. While it may (or may not) have helped control the child's fever, did it cause liver damage? In September 2002, the Food and Drug Administration Nonprescription Advisory Board reported that acetaminophen can cause liver damage and failure. Therefore, no one should take more than the recommended dose of acetaminophen and for no longer than four days (FDA consumer, 2003). In fact, a finding of a 2005 study found that overdose of the painkiller acetaminophen is the leading cause of acute liver failure in the United States (Healthfacts, 2006).

5. Does this make sense for my patient population?

If you find the results of a study farfetched and vastly opposed to your experience and current practice, read the study with caution. You do not need to include every research study done on a topic for evidence in your EBP project. This is particularly so if the evidence found does not match the age or sex of your patient population. Always ask yourself, "Does this make sense?"

These are some basic questions to ask when looking at the results of a research study. Now, let's look more closely at the actual components of the research study report. A simple worksheet to evaluate a research study is given in the appendix to this chapter. Let's break down each component that is addressed on the worksheet.

Key areas to examine when critiquing a research study article.

1. *What type of study is the research article?*
   Is it quantitative or qualitative
2. *What are the qualifications of the person who did the research?*
   Is the person qualified to do the study? For example, if you are evaluating a research article on children's pain levels and the researcher never worked with children and does not routinely assess pain in practice, he or she would not be qualified. Another example is if you are evaluating a research article about educating student nurses. It would make sense if the researcher were a professor or someone who understands and works with nursing students.
3. *The title*
   Does the title describe what the research study is about? Is the title short and concise, or long and convoluted? For example, suppose you are reviewing a research article about

children's reaction to stress in the hospital. You see the title of the article is, "How do adults respond to stress?" This would not be appropriate for your EBP because it does not mention the patient population involved in your research study, which is children.

4. *Abstract*

The abstract is the summary of all points of the study. It should contain enough information to enable you to evaluate key aspects of the study? The abstract should contain the **purpose, research question(s), method,** and **major findings of the study?** Does it contain these items, and does it summarize the results of the study? What is the exact method or process the researcher(s) went through to conduct the study? How was the study done? Is the topic interesting and relevant to your patient population or problem of interest of your EBP project?

5. *Introduction*

An introductory paragraph should always be given. This paragraph should not only present the topic, but grab your interest and provide a brief overview of the topic at hand. What is the research problem? Basically, what is the point of the study? Has the researcher appropriately described the scope of the problem? Does the problem have significance for the nursing profession? How will the research contribute to nursing practice, nursing administration, and/ or nursing education? Is the problem to be addressed formally presented as a statement of purpose, research question, or hypothesis to be tested? Is this information communicated clearly and concisely?

6. *Purpose*

The purpose of the study should always be stated. It is very important to understand the motivation of researchers and how they feel their research study will forward either nursing science or nursing care. If it is a not a nursing-based research study, it should still explain what purpose it hopes to serve in the healthcare environment.

7. *Research questions*

Every research study should have a research question or questions as a guide. What are the questions the researcher hopes to answer? It is important to note that these questions are not the same thing as the purpose of the study. The research question(s) should fulfill the purpose, but are not the same as the purpose.

8. *Hypothesis*

All quantitative research studies have a hypothesis or prediction of what the researcher thinks is going to happen. By developing a hypothesis, researchers are better able to identify possible sources of their own bias. Most often when researchers conduct research, they have a "feeling" or indication of how the study will turn out. Now, they may either be trying to prove their hypothesis correct or prove their hypothesis or prediction incorrect. This is an important part of the research study process. It is also important that the hypothesis makes sense for the study as well. It would make no sense to make a prediction that cannot even be proven by the research study at hand. If the report does not formally state any hypotheses, is the reason stated? Do the hypotheses (if any) flow from a theory or previous research? If not, what is the basis for the researcher's predictions? Are the hypotheses (if any) properly worded (i.e., do they state a predicted relationship between two or more variables)? Is there a rationale for the manner in which they were stated? Are hypotheses stated as research hypotheses or null hypotheses?

Fast facts in a nutshell

Remember that qualitative studies do not have a hypothesis or test a hypothesis as do quantitative studies. In qualitative studies, the goal is to understand a phenomenon as it naturally exists in the world and to identify common themes. Predictions of outcome are not made. The qualitative researcher uses broad research questions to guide the study and seeks to understand meaningful patterns which evolve.

9. *Literature Review*

An extensive review of the literature should be completed. It is important to view all research done on a given topic before embarking on any future research. You need to "know where we've been, to know where we are going or plan to go." The literature review should include relevant research studies, particularly within the last five years. If older studies are included, their importance should be explained. If they are landmark studies, propose significant changes, or reflect discoveries in the area being researched, include them. Confirm that the coverage of the literature seems thorough and complete? Does it appear that the review includes all or most of the major studies that have been conducted on the topic of interest? Are recent research reports cited? How recent are the reports? Does the review rely on appropriate materials (i.e., mainly on research reports, using primary or secondary sources)? Is the review organized so that development of ideas is clear? If the review is part of a research report for a new study, does the review support the need for the new research? If the review is designed to guide clinical practice, does the review support the need for (or lack of need for) changes in practice? Does the review conclude with a synopsis of the state-of-the-art knowledge on the topic? Is the style of the review appropriate? Does the reviewer paraphrase or is there an overreliance on quotations? Does the review appear unbiased? Does the reviewer use appropriate language? Does the review flow logically?

Fast facts in a nutshell

Keep in mind that the length of time between the time research is completed and the time it is published in a scholarly journal may be up to two years. Therefore, much of the most recent research articles are outdated before they are published. The time varies from journal to journal.

---

10. **Ethical aspects of the study**

    When examining a research study, you want to be sure that the study was conducted ethically, especially if you want to use the study for "evidence." No study participants should ever be subjected to any physical harm, discomfort, or psychological distress. The researchers must take appropriate steps to remove them from and keep them from being harmed. It is important when doing research to consider if the research benefit to participants in the study outweighs any potential risk to them. In addition, consider if the benefits to society outweigh the costs to the participants. No type of coercion or undue influence should be used in recruiting or selecting the participants. When working with vulnerable subjects, special considerations need to be observed. The participants should never be deceived or tricked in any way to participate in the study. They must be made fully aware that they are participating in a study. You should ensure that they understand the purpose of the study and why the research is being done. Informed consent must always be obtained. Privacy and confidentiality must also be taken to protect the participants. Lastly, when a research study is conducted in an institution, such as a hospital, the research must be approved and monitored by an Institutional Review Board (IRB) or other similar ethics review committee.

Fast facts in a nutshell

Vulnerable subjects are people who are not capable of giving a fully informed consent. This could be the result of mental incapacity or age. Examples of vulnerable subjects are children, mentally challenged or emotionally disabled people, someone in a coma, severely or terminally ill people, and pregnant women. Note that pregnant women can give informed consent, but the unborn fetus cannot. The risk to the unborn fetus must be examined, and the risk-benefit ratio for the pregnant mother and for the fetus must be weighed heavily when embarking on a research study. This is documented in the Code of Federal Regulations, 2005 which can be viewed at http://www.hhs.gov/ohrp/humansubjects/guidance/45cfr46.htm

11. **Conceptual and theoretical frameworks**

    A conceptual or theoretical framework guides the study. Remember the theory or conceptual model does not have to come only from the field of nursing. It can be from another discipline, such as psychology. But consider if a relevant conceptual or theoretical framework was used for the study? Does it flow? Does the framework make sense for the type of study? Is it explained clearly?

12. **Operational terms**

    Operational terms are terms that may have different meanings when used in different contexts, so the study should explain how such words will be defined. Thus, you want to see if operational terms are used. You also want to know if the term and definition is appropriate for the given study and if they help to clarify exactly what the term means in the study. They are simply definitions of the words and how each will be used in the study.

13. **Research Design**

    What is the basic type of design? Remember the two main types of research, quantitative or qualitative. Within each of these categories, what type of design is used for the study? For example, is a quantitative study experimental or nonexperimental? Remember in an experimental, comparative, or randomized study, the study is divided into two groups. One group is experimental and receives the experimental drug, therapy, treatment, or intervention, while the second group does not receive it. Keep in mind that random assignment is necessary for experimental studies. If studies are randomly assigned, the results are more credible and can be generalized to other similar studies (Carlson, Kruse & Rouse, 1999). In addition, examine is if there are variables. If so, how do they affect each other? Name the basic type of design to help your understanding of the content of the research. See Chapters 4 and 5 for further clarification of the different types of research. Always remember to check if any bias is present the study? Are there influences present that may affect the results?

Fast facts in a nutshell

Validity is the ability to measure what is supposed to be measured. In research studies, an inference is made or reasons/causes and a rationale are given describing the study results (the effect). Threats to validity are the reasons why a study may contain incorrect inferences. The researcher should try to control threats to validity in any study. Remember that it is hard to control 100% of everything or every outcome in a study, but the researcher must try to control as many variables as he or she can.

14. **Population and sample**

    How were the subjects or participants for the study selected? Was randomization used?

    Quantitative Sampling Designs. Is the population identified, described, and easily accessible? Are eligibility criteria clearly described? Are the sample selection procedures clearly described? What type of sampling plan was used? Does the sample adequately represent the total population? Did some factor affect the representativeness of the sample (i.e., a low response rate)? Are possible sample biases identified? Is the sample size sufficiently large or too small?

    Qualitative Sampling Designs. Is the setting adequately described? Is the setting and population appropriate for the research question(s)? How were the participants selected for the study? Was the sampling approach appropriate? Is the sample size adequate, too small or too large? Did the researcher state that information saturation was achieved?

15. **Data collection methods?**

    Who collected the research data? Were the data collectors qualified for this role or is there something about them (e.g., their professional role, their relationship with study participants) that could undermine the collection of unbiased, high-quality data? How were data collectors trained? Does the training appear adequate? Where and under what circumstances were the data gathered? Were other people present during the data collection? Could the presence of others have created any influence or bias? Did the collection of data place any undue burdens (in terms of time or stress) on participants? How might this have affected data quality?

Fast facts in a nutshell

Interrater reliability is a term used when you have two or more individuals or "coders" gathering information during a study. It is the degree to which they agree. For judging purposes, it is a consensus; it is how often they agree on a given score. In research, it is how often two observers agree on a given item and the level of agreement between them. This is very important in research when more than one person is gathering the data.

---

16. **Statistical significance**
    Were the collected data statistically significant? All the data in the world could be collected but if they are not statistically significant, they are meaningless. It is very important to achieve statistical significance. The two easiest ways of understanding statistical significance is to look at the "p value" and the confidence interval. Review Chapter 4 for a further explanation of statistical significance and these concepts.
17. **Significance for your area of practice**
    Most important when evaluating evidence is to ask yourself this question, "Is this information significant to my patient population or evidence-based practice project?" If it is not, then discard it; if it is, keep it for "evidence."

18. **Assumptions and Limitations**

    Assumptions are presuppositions that the researcher makes about the study before it begins. This is what the researcher is "taking for granted," so to speak. For example, the researcher assumes people will want to participate in the study.

    Limitations prevent the study from reaching its full potential. For example, the researcher wanted to study the effects of sunshine on people's happiness, but it rained for the duration of the study. Another example would be if the researcher wanted to study 10-year-old boys, but only two 10-year-old boys were available. These limitations should be discussed and presented.

19. **Conclusions**

    Do you agree with the conclusions the author drew from the study? In your opinion, did the author(s) draw incorrect conclusions or jump to conclusions not easily made from the evidence?

20. **Implications for future research**

    Does the author or researcher explain the implications of the findings for future research? These implications are areas identified by the researcher for further exploration and research. These are ideas another researcher may choose to pursue. These are also areas a new or novice researcher could use when embarking on a research project. Reviewing the research literature and EBP may indeed uncover other areas that may be in need of future or further research.

Summary

You should ask yourself the basic questions given above when reviewing evidence for your EBP. This worksheet does not list all questions that should be asked, but it does give the novice a good basis for evaluating research studies. In addition, researchers should review the guidelines for critiquing quantitative and qualitative studies (see Table 4.2 and Table 5,3).

In a research study, French (2006) found that specialist nurses use two main criteria, relevance and quality, to evaluate research in practice. Other criteria given in order of frequency were effectiveness, practicality, impact, effort, staff, and feasibility. *Effectiveness* meant whether the intervention was going to do what it what intended to do. *Practicality* meant whether implementation of an intervention was functional, efficient, or sufficient in meeting the purpose for which it was intended. *Impact* described the patient reacted to the intervention, and whether the intervention could cause a patient any harm. *Effort* related to how easy it would be to implement the intervention. *Staff* was how nurses would be affected by implementing the intervention. *Feasibility* was the last and most consistent criterion examined. How difficult or feasible would it be to implement this nursing intervention. You will probably relate to these criteria when examining evidence to determine whether to recommend implementation of an intervention in your practice area.

In a second research study, Sandelowski and Barroso (2002) examined how to isolate the findings in qualitative research, as sometimes the data is misrepresented as findings. This means that some data is presented that may not be findings that relate to the study at hand. In addition, reports sometimes contain very little description to support the researcher's interpretations of the data. For example, how does the researcher eliminate their own biases in the interpretation of the data? Quotations and descriptions of incidents may be misused. Excessive quoting of participants may be included, but they may not fit with the purpose of the study or the conclusions obtained. Researchers also sometimes do not state how they came up with patterns or themes. Finally, conceptual conclusions or theories that are used may drift from one concept to another and not truly represent the theory given as a basis for a study. These are some of the challenges given by Sandelowski and Barroso (2002) in locating and evaluating the findings in qualitative research articles. So, if you become confused in determining what is good or bad research, do not hesitate to consult a person with more experience critiquing research. This can be a colleague, a professor at a local college, or someone in your institution's research department.

Fast Facts in a nutshell

When rating evidence for EBP, the highest level of evidence is that from a systematic review or metaanalysis of all relevant randomized controlled trials (RCTs) or established EBP clinical guidelines.

THE STRENGTH OF THE EVIDENCE

How strong is the evidence being used? What level of research is being used? There are numerous ways to grade or evaluate research evidence for use in EBP. The Agency for Healthcare Research and Quality (AHRQ) is a federally funded agency that supports quality-of-care and evidence-based practice through Evidence-Based Practice Centers (EBPCs) across the United States. The U.S. Preventative Services Task Force (USPSTF), which is supported by AHRQ, evaluates scientific studies related to clinical preventative services and makes recommendations based on specific criteria. These recommendations allow clinicians to make informed practice decisions. This task force grades the evidence as: "A" (strongly recommends), "B" (recommends), "C" (no recommendation for or against), "D" (recommends against), or "I" (insufficient evidence to recommend for or against). The evidence is graded on quality, quantity, and consistency (Long, 2009). More information about this system can be obtained at http://www. ahrq.gov/CLINIC/uspstfix.htm.

The AHRQ recently supported a study in which 121 systems designed to rate evidence were evaluated to determine "best practice" in this area. The results identified gaps in rating quality, strength of evidence, and application of these grading schemes to the less traditional types of research, such as observational studies. The authors concluded that there is not (nor will there be in the near future) a single system that can be used to grade scholarly work across all disciplines. They also concluded that evidence gathering differs from clinician to clinician. These results show the difficulty in determining exactly what is evidence and how it might best be applied to practice (Malloch & Porter O'Grady, 2005). For more information about this study and current recommendations, see http://www.ahrq.gov/Clinic/epcix.htm.

One of the most common evidence ratings systems in nursing was put forth by Melnyk & Fineout-Overholt (2005). It is the evidence hierarchy shown in Table 7.2.

Another way to evaluate your evidence is according the GRADE rating hierarchy to see which of your research articles offers the strongest type of evidence available (see Table 7.2). Although several evidence ranking and grading schemes exist, controversy over which one is best led to an international effort to develop a universal system of evaluation. In 2000, an informal collaboration of people addressed the shortcomings

TABLE 7.2   Rating System for Hierarchy of Evidence

Level 1:   Evidence from a systematic review or metaanalysis of all relevant randomized controlled trials (RCTs) or evidence-based clinical practice guidelines based on systematic reviews of RCTs and EBP clinical guidelines.

Level 2:   Evidence obtained from at least one well-designed RCT.

Level 3:   Evidence obtained from a well-designed controlled trial without randomization.

Level 4:   Evidence from well-designed case-control and cohort studies.

Level 5:   Evidence from systematic reviews of descriptive and qualitative studies.

Level 6:   Evidence from a single descriptive or qualitative study.

Level 7:   Evidence from the opinion of authorities and/or reports of expert Committees.

From Melynk, Fineout-Overholt (2005). Reprinted with permission from Lippincott, Williams & Wilkins.

and the multiple evidence grading systems in health care. This international system is known as GRADE, which stands for grades of recommendation, assessment, development, and evaluation. The GRADE system ranks evidence into four levels: 1) high, 2) moderate, 3) low, and 4) very low. The recommendation is either 1) strong or 2) weak (Long, 2009). You can learn more about the GRADE system at http://www.gradeworkinggroup.org/FAQ/index.htm.

Sometimes it is helpful to have a tool to critique studies when you are first starting out. Please see the appendix to this chapter for an example of a tool you can use.

Fast facts in a nutshell: summary

In summary, critiquing the evidence can be very confusing. You should know how to ask questions and review important aspects of the evidence and research reports you find. Understand how to grade the evidence and how to determine what makes evidence strong or weak. Efforts have been undertaken by various groups to make a uniform system of evidence evaluation, so that research is being graded or evaluated in the same way.

REFERENCES

Barone, S., Roy, C., & Frederickson, K. (2008). Instruments used in Roy adaptation Model-based research: Review, critique and further directions. Nursing Science Quarterly, 21(4), 353–362.

Carlton, D. S., Kruse, L. K., & Rouse, C. L. (1999). The research column: Critiquing nursing research. A user friendly guide for the staff nurse. Journal of Emergency Nursing, 25(4), 330–332.

Federal Drug Administration (FDA). (2003). Use caution with pain relievers, FDA Consumer, 37(1), 36.

French, B. (2006). Evaluating research for use in practice: What criteria do specialist nurses use? Journal of Advanced Nursing, 50(3), 235–243.

Healthfacts (2006). Overdose of acetaminophen, AKA Tylenol, The leading cause of acute liver failure in the U.S. Healthfacts, 31(4), 2–3.

Kolcaba, K. (2008). Comfort theory. Retrieved July 10, 2009 from http://www.thecomfortline.com/comfort_theory.html

Long, C. O. (2009). Weighing in on the evidence. In N. Schmidt & J. Brown (Eds.), Evidence-based practice for nurses: Appraisal and application of research. Boston: Jones & Bartlett.

Malloch, K., & Porter O'Grady, T. (2005). Evidence-based practice in nursing and healthcare. Sudbury, MA: Jones & Barltett

Melnyk, B. M., & Fineout-Overholt, E. (2005) Evidence-based practice in nursing and health care: A guide to best practice. Philadelphia: Lippincott, Williams & Wilkins.

Polit, D. F., & Beck, C. T. (2008). Nursing research: Generating and assessing evidence for nursing practice (8th ed.). Philadelphia: Lippincott, Williams & Wilkins.

Polit D. F., & Beck, C. T. (2005). Essentials of nursing research (6th ed.). Philadelphia: Lippincott, Williams & Wilkins.

Sandelowski, M., & Barroso, J. (2002). Finding the findings in qualitative studies. Journal of Nursing Scholarship, 34(3), 213–219.

Chapter 7 Appendix

Article Critique Worksheet

When critiquing a research article, answer the following questions by filling in the blank or circling your response.

1. Is the study **quantitative** or **qualitative?**

2. Is the **researcher qualified?** (yes or no) Why or why not?

_____

_____

_____

3. **Title-** appropriate? (yes or no) Clear and concise? (yes or no)

4. **Abstract**
   - Is the hypothesis or research question present and list it.

_____

_____

_____

- What is the method of research?

_____

_____

_____

- Is a description of the findings present?

_____

_____

_____

- Are the major findings listed? If so what are they?

_____

_____

_____

5. **Introduction**
   - Introductory paragraph? (yes or no)
   - Does the introduction grab your interest? (yes or no)
   - Any background information? (yes or no)
   (Is the significance to nursing stated? (yes or no)

6. **Purpose:** What is the purpose of this research article?

_____

_____

_____

7. **Research problem:** Is the research problem identified? (yes or no) What is it?

_____

_____

_____

8. **Hypothesis**
   - Is the hypothesis stated? (yes or no) What is it?

   _____

   _____

   _____

   - Do you think the hypothesis makes sense (is a good guess) for the given study? (yes or no) Why or why not?

   _____

   _____

   _____

9. **Literature review**
   - How many articles are reviewed by the author and listed in the reference section? _____
   - Is it an adequate number in your opinion? (yes or no)
   - Are the resources relevant to the topic being studied? (yes or no)
   - Are the resources current? (yes or no)
   - How many resources given were published within the last 5 years? _____
     the last 10 years _____ older than 10 years _____

10. **Ethical considerations**
    Were ethical practices used when conducting the study? (yes or no)
    If not, what was done in the study that you would consider unethical?

    _____

    _____

    _____

11. **Theoretical or conceptual framework**
    - Was a framework present or not? (yes or no) If yes, can you identify it?

    _____

    _____

    _____

    - What type of theory or framework was used?

    _____

    _____

    _____

    - Was this theory or framework from the field of nursing? (yes or no)

12. **Operational terms**
    - Are there operational terms given? (yes or no)
    - Are the terms appropriate for the given study? (yes or no)
    - Do they help clarify the study? (yes or no) Why or why not?

    _____

    _____

    _____

13. **Research design**
    - We have already classified if the main type of research is quantitative or qualitative. Within that main classification, what type of research is it? (i.e. experimental or nonexperimental, phenomenological, etc).

    _____

    _____

    _____

- What is the method used to assign subjects?

_____

_____

_____

- Was there randomization? (yes or no)
- Are there any variables? If so, list them below:
  variable 1:

_____

_____

_____

  variable 2:

_____

_____

_____

  variable 3:

_____

_____

_____

  variable 4:

_____

_____

_____

- Is there any bias present and, if so, list what you
  think is biased.

_____

_____

_____

- If the study has bias, think about who funded the study, Who conducted the study? Where do they work? Is there a conflict of interest present?

_____

_____

_____

14. **Population and sample**
    - Who was studied?

_____

_____

_____

   - What was the age group?

_____

_____

_____

   - How many people were studied or used? What is the exact sample size?
     $n = $ _____

   - Do you think this is an adequate sample size? (yes or no) Why or why not?

_____

_____

_____

15. What was the **data collection method?** (survey, questionnaire, etc.)

_____

_____

_____

16. Was the study **statistically significant?**
    • What are the **p values?**

_____

_____

_____

    • What is the **confidence interval?**

_____

_____

_____

17. Was this study significant to the field of nursing? (yes or no) Why or why not?

_____

_____

_____

18. **Assumptions/limitations**
    • Did the author list any assumptions? (yes or no) If yes, what were they?

_____

_____

_____

    • Did the author list any limitations (yes or no) If yes, what were they?

_____

_____

_____

19. **Conclusions:** What were the conclusions?

_____

_____

_____

20. **Implications for future research.** Where there any implications or suggestions for future areas of research given by the author? (yes or no) If so what are they, and do you find them sensible and appropriate?

_____

_____

_____

_____

_____

_____

_____

_____

Chapter 8

Barriers to Disseminating the Evidence

INTRODUCTION

This chapter examines some of the barriers to conducting research and implementing evidence-based practice (EBP) projects in nursing. Sometimes, fear of the unknown and the effects of peer pressure, along with strong nursing traditions, are the main reasons for inhibiting the development of an evidence-based practice environment. In addition, organizational constraints, such as lack of administrative support or incentives to move forward with evidence-based practice, are explored. Finally, the chapter discusses how to overcome some of these obstacles.

In this chapter, you will learn:

1. The barriers to implementing EBP.
2. How to change your practice environment.
3. How technology affects EBP research.
4. Ways to disseminate or present EBP research.

BARRIERS TO SUCCESSFUL RESEARCH AND IMPLEMENTATION OF EBP

Chapter 1 mentioned the following barriers to successful research:

- Lack of awareness or understanding of EBP.
- Lack of association with researchers.
- Lack of ability to locate or find relevant research.
- Lack of ability to "understand the language" of research.
- Lack of the value of research in nursing practice.
- Lack of availability of computer databases.
- Lack of basic knowledge of information technology.
- Lack of time to obtain research information.

These barriers are very real in the practice environment today. We must explore ways to eliminate them, so that nursing can move forward as a profession. Patient-centered care requires that we practice nursing using the latest and best evidence to provide the best care possible for our patients. Collaboration with physicians and other healthcare practitioners is vital to building a collegial relationship based on trust, respect, and the best evidence. We must never tire of trying to find ways to implement EBP.

Australia and the United Kingdom have been leaders in the implementation of EBP. In the United States in nursing, EBP is increasingly being implemented. The move of hospital institutions to "Magnet status" could potentially be the impetus for this change. Magnet status is an award given by the American Nurses' Credentialing Center (ANCC), an affiliate of the American Nurses Association, to hospitals that satisfy a set of criteria designed to measure the strength and quality of their nursing staffs. **A Magnet hospital is one in which nursing results in excellent patient outcomes, where nurses have a high level of job satisfaction, and where there is a low staff nurse turnover rate and appropriate grievance resolution.** Magnet status also indicates nurse involvement in data collection and decision-making in patient care delivery. The idea is that Magnet nursing leaders value staff nurses, involve them in shaping research-based nursing practice, and encourage and reward them for advancing in nursing practice. Magnet hospitals are supposed to have open communication between nurses and other members of the healthcare team, and an appropriate personnel mix to attain the best patient outcomes and staff work environment (Center for Nursing Advocacy, 2007). This is accomplished by examining the current research trends and incorporating them into practice.

Fast facts in a nutshell

A Magnet hospital is one in which nursing results in excellent patient outcomes, where nurses have a high level of job satisfaction, and where there is a low staff nurse turnover rate and appropriate grievance resolution

But what do you do if the institution you work at is a smaller agency or does not have Magnet status? Where do you start to attract interest for EBP?

It is wise to first assess what the particular barriers are to EBP in your facility. You might accomplish this by a simple informal survey. A focus group also might be used, which is a small group of individuals who meet together and are asked questions by a moderator about a particular topic and then discuss the topic at hand. For example, the topic could be one's knowledge base, attitudes and beliefs, and thoughts regarding the research process and how to use research or evidence in practice. In addition, determine to what level staff members believe that implementing EBP will result in improved patient care or better outcomes. **If healthcare practitioners do not believe that EBP will result in improved care and patient outcomes, the facilitator needs to provide examples or real-case scenarios of how this would occur.** This is how a focus group works. In addition, by providing examples, particularly ones where cost savings could occur, administrators may well be more willing to consider implementing EBP. For example, if you work in a private nursing home and you are trying to implement an environment of EBP, you might use the latest research to show that the use of an incontinent device that initially costs a dollar more than the old device could eventually save hundreds of dollars in linen services, decubitus care, and better outcomes for the patient. This proposal may definitely be taken under closer consideration. Using EBP to provide cost savings is usually always well received by administrators. It is paramount for nurses to articulate the value of interventions within an economic framework to maintain institutional viability.

Fast facts in a nutshell

If healthcare practitioners do not believe that EBP will result in improved care and patient outcomes, the facilitator needs to provide examples or real-case scenarios of how this would occur.

CHANGING THE PRACTICE ENVIRONMENT

One cannot ignore today's issues of nursing availability, productivity, working conditions, and the aging of the nursing workforce. With nurses in short supply, many healthcare systems are struggling with the issue of a nursing shortage. The hospital restructuring movement in the early 1990s resulted in reductions in the educated nursing workforce, ultimately threatening the clinical viability of the organization at the same time that clinical interventions were becoming more complex. These productivity decisions made in the early to mid-1990s have taken a large toll on the nursing resources in healthcare systems today. The historic lack of connection between the economic viability of the organization and the satisfaction and performance of the nursing resources is a very important factor to consider in looking to the future viability of healthcare organizations. **Nurses are indeed at the "crossroads of care" in the healthcare organization.** It is the nurses' role to be the "eyes of the physician" and to quickly evaluate, coordinate, integrate, and facilitate all of the clinical functions related to the delivery of patient care. While this is a vital function of the nurse, the nurse must also recognize that he or she should evaluate the evidence of clinical practice that delivers optimal patient outcomes. This is where nursing must take the lead and be proactive. The process of reframing nursing calls for nurses to critically evaluate both its clinical foundations and support the financial demands faced by the healthcare institution. This is where nursing can make a difference. Evidence-based practice is one method to improve patient outcomes. This takes the nurse from a previous focus only on the clinical process to a new focus that requires paying attention to clinical outcomes (Malloch & Porter-O'Grady, 2006).

Fast facts in a nutshell

Nurses are indeed at the "crossroads of care" in the healthcare organization. It is the nurse's role to be the "eyes of the physician" and to quickly evaluate, coordinate, integrate, and facilitate all of the clinical functions related to the delivery of patient care.

TECHNOLOGY, DATABASES, AND EVIDENCE-BASED PRACTICE

It is imperative that the latest and best evidence be incorporated into EBP. This is done by having access to the databases that contain the information or latest research studies that can affect care. If the institution in which you work provides access to scientific databases, that is excellent. If it does not, you need to obtain information about accessing the databases and the cost to acquire them. Then provide that information to the leaders or managers of your institution. Again, some of the services, such as Science Direct, EBSCO, OVID provide several databases for a fee. There are bundle packages available to purchase. These services are indeed expensive for the smaller institutions, but an argument must be made for how these databases will support the infrastructure of research and advancing science in your institution. **Make an argument for evidence based practice.** You might also make an argument for a joint venture to purchase these on-line full text databases between departments or institutions to decrease the cost to an individual institution. Remember that some of the journals contained in the databases require that content not be made available electronically for a year. So, it may be wise to subscribe to important research journals or realize that most often you can go directly to the journal's Web site and access for free the most recent issue. There are also "**e-zines**" or "**e-journals**" that are available on the internet. These are simply electronic versions of the journal and articles contained in them.

LACK OF KNOWLEDGE ABOUT EVIDENCE-BASED PRACTICE

It is vital that classes are offered to educate the staff about EBP. Sometimes, a lack of knowledge about EBP or fear of the unknown is the single most important barrier to convincing colleagues to get on board and understand the process. In a

2002 study, Jolly noted that nurses' attitudes toward research and development were poor until a program was developed to assist them in understanding how to read and critically appraise research articles. Programs or classes may be held as formal or informal in-service education learning to assist in this process. Many fear the process of searching for research articles. This text and your support should, however, prove invaluable in alleviating their fears. Encourage peers to visit databases, such as the *Cochrane Library* and the *National Guidelines Clearinghouse,* which can provide quick and already completed systematic reviews and EBP guidelines for implementation. Check your local colleges and universities for courses about EBP. There are also on-line resources that are run by nursing schools that can serve as a resource for learning about EBP. Many of these are selected centers that have developed around the world with the primary purpose of promoting EBP (see Table 8-1).

Melnyk & Fineout-Overholt (2005), state that little research has been done on developing and sustaining EBP. Forty-four systematic reviews focusing on the effects of strategies to change practice of healthcare professionals were located and analyzed. The following conclusions were drawn:

- Passive dissemination of research is ineffective.
- A range of intervention has been shown to be effective in changing the behavior of healthcare professionals.
- Multifaceted interventions are more likely to be effective than a single intervention.
- Individual practitioners' beliefs, attitudes, and knowledge influence their behavior, but other factors, including orga-

TABLE 8.1   Online Resources for Tutorials for EBP

The Academic Center for Evidence-Based Nursing at the University of Texas Health Science Center at San Antonio.
http://www.acestart.uthscsa.edu/

The Center for Health Evidence
http://www.cche.net/usersguides/main.asp

Johanna Briggs Institute for Evidence-Based Nursing and Midwifery
http://www.joannabriggs.edu.au

The Center for Research & Evidence-Based Practice at the University of Rochester School of Nursing in New York
www.urmc.rochester.edu/son/ebp/

University of Rochester Medical Center, Edward G. Miner Library. Evidence Based Practice Tutorial
http://www.urmc.rochester.edu/hslt/miner/resources/evidence_based/index.cfm
http://www.urmc.rochester.edu/Miner/Links/ebmlinks.html

The Sara Cole Hirsch Institute for Best Nursing Practice Based on Evidence at Case Western Reserve School of Nursing
http://fpb.case.edu/HirshInstitute/index.shtm

Students guide to medical literature
http://grinch.uchsc.edu/sg//index.html

nizational, economic, and community environments, also are important.

* A diagnostic analysis should be conducted to identify barriers and supportive factors likely to influence the proposed change in practice.
* Successful strategies to change practice need to be adequately resourced and require people with appropriate knowledge and skills.

Since there are such diverse personalities, health professionals, and clinical settings, it is important to involve more resource and support, as well as a paradigm and culture shift in the organization. Strategies suggested by Melnyk & Fineout-Overholt (2005) are:

* One-on-one sessions between health professional educators and individual staff to explain the desired practice change or the concepts of EBP.
* Manual and computerized reminders to prompt the practitioner behavior change in practice.
* Educational meetings or in-services that require active participation of the learners.
* Audits and feedback in which clinical performance is monitored through electronic database or chart review.
* Direct observation and feedback.

In addition, the author supports:

* The involvement of unit-based committees, such as performance improvement (PI), quality assurance (QA), or pol-

icy and procedure committee members to facilitate the EBP process.

- Journal or research article clubs that enhance the discussion of a particular article per month. Several studies (McQueen et al., 2006; Karkos & Peters, 2006; Wilson & Collins, 2005; Jolly, 2002) have found that journal clubs increased awareness, knowledge, confidence, and skills in research.
- Poster presentations in which each unit in an institution shares with the entire healthcare institution ideas and EBP projects created, on-going, or developed by each unit.
- Nursing research day with presentations and seminars to encourage participation and facilitate understanding of EBP.

OFFERING INCENTIVES

Incentives are always a motivating factor to bring about interest and change in the workplace environment. Contests can be arranged with prizes given. Provide food for free for attendance at any EBP program. Free t-shirts, bookbags, or pen give-a-ways are a nice way to generate interest and increase attendance. A simple gift of a chocolate bar for attendance would suffice as a motivational factor for some. Survey the population you will be working with and provide incentives of interest to that group.

INCLUDING EVIDENCE-BASED PRACTICE IN PERFORMANCE APPRAISALS

Another idea that managers can use to implement and facilitate environmental change is to require involvement in EBP as part of the annual performance appraisal. Many times a monetary motivation tied to the annual performance appraisal can be a great motivating force to move staff toward involvement in the EBP process.

TIME AND SUPPORT

Most importantly, administrators must realize that they cannot expect nurses to "fit" research and EBP into the normal daily care rituals. Most know the rigor and demands of the clinical work environment and time away from the job must be allotted to encourage participation and interest. Administrative support for this process is vital. It is well worth the time to present the EBP process to the management and enlist the support of the administration before embarking on the EBP process.

DISSEMINATING THE EVIDENCE

Once you have gained interest and support for EBP, new and exciting projects can be planned and implemented. Do not forget to share your results with colleagues. So much of the wonderful work done in nursing is never published or shared. Below are a few ways that we can share the wonderful work we do in moving the science of nursing forward.

Oral Presentations

Present EBP projects and successful implementation strategies at local conferences, national conferences, or intrahospital in-services.

PRESENTING EVIDENCE-BASED PRACTICE INFORMATION

When presenting the information you have developed about an EBP project, be both systematic and organized. Most conference presentations are approximately 20 to 30 minutes. When planning a presentation, be clear and concise. If presenting PowerPoint slides, be sure that the type on the slides is at least 28 point in the selected font, so that attendees can read them clearly from the back of the room. You should also use sharp and contrasting colors that are easily read in a large room. Use white when writing on black background and white when writing on a black background. Avoid the overuse of clip art or pictures that will detract from your professional presentation.

To organize your content, start by making an outline. **Start every presentation with objectives or a list of the outcomes you want the learner to achieve.** Then clearly present your EBP project. You can follow the steps below:

1. Introduce your clinical problem or EBP topic.
2. State the purpose you hoped to achieve with your project or problem of interest. What is it that you wanted to change in practice, or what inspired you to examine this topic?
3. Include any theoretical or conceptual frameworks that may have guided your work (not usually used in EBP, but more so in a nursing research project).
4. What interventions did you implement or examine in your EBP project?
5. **Provide a brief summary of "the evidence."** This can be done in a table format written in American Psychological Association (APA) format. You may also want to include

the ranking or hierarchy of evidence (e.g., randomized controlled trial (RCT), level 1 or highest and strongest type of evidence. You may also want to include acceptable clinical practice guidelines already established.

6. What did you find in conducting your project that lead to or did not lead to a practice change? This is a summary of your findings. Also include what implications this will have for future practice or research possibilities needed.

This presentation can be done live in a conference setting, live in an institutional or clinical setting, or as a poster presentation. More information about these methods will be presented later in this chapter.

Panel Discussions

Panel discussions are sometimes used to share and discuss the findings of EBP issues or research. The panel is usually a group of experts in the field. Before the discussion, determine the allotted amount of time for each speaker and which speaker will handle which topic. Remember to allow a question-and-answer period to encourage the audience to participate in the discussion. This can be done in a professional conference setting or informally in an institutional or clinical setting.

Poster Presentations

Poster presentations are probably the easiest way to disseminate current nursing information. Poster presentations may be given at local or national conferences. Sharing information at a national conference provides important and timely information for colleagues and practitioners. The methods of composing and sharing the poster are different depending on the type of organization sponsoring the event. Be sure to find out the criteria for submitting an abstract of a poster before sending any information. In addition, be sure to find out the actual poster criteria before making the poster. Many conferences have size requirements and may or may not provide instruments to hang the poster if needed. The typical size for a poster is 4 feet by 6 feet. It is also important to plan the graphics and pictures incorporated in a poster. The golden rule is for the attendee at the conference to be able to view the poster from four feet away. Some other items to consider in presenting a poster are listed below:

- Consider the audience attending the conference, including the language of the attendees. Do the members speak primarily English? Are they professional medical people or laypeople. If laypeople, medical jargon may be confusing to them.
- Make the poster readable. Vary the size of the font used in the poster. Do not make the letters too small or too large or they will detract from the content of the poster. The conference attendee should be able to read the poster highlights from a foot away.
- Use pictures or graphics only when they add to the content of your poster. A few graphics are eye pleasing if they are relevant, but too many graphics make the poster "busy" and can frustrate the reader.
- Use a font that is easy to read. Consider the typical fonts you use to write a paper, such as Times New Roman or Arial. Use

the same font throughout the poster. You can use a special or decorative font, such as comic sans at a pediatric conference, if it is appropriate for the type of conference.

- Avoid shadowing the letters. This can make the letters hard to read.
- Consider providing attendees with handouts that summarize your poster and provide your contact information. You can also distribute business cards that attendees can take to their own practice environment and share with their colleagues. These handouts can be in color or black and white. The handouts can be an outline of your information or a copy of the poster itself. Consider cost when making handouts. Color is obviously more expensive.
- Be present at your poster during schedule poster/exhibit times to answer questions conference attendees may have. This also gives you a time to network with other professionals in your practice area.

Small Group Presentations

The results of your EBP study can be shared in small groups at a multitude of places. This can be done among a few (3-6) of your peers or colleagues over a lunch or dinner break; on the clinical unit or in a classroom or auditorium; through a grand-rounds type presentation; through professional committee meetings (either unit-based or hospital or institutional-wide); or, if relevant, in the community or at a comparable agency or worksite.

Professional Publications

Did you ever wonder who writes the articles in the journals you read? The answer is people just like you. If you develop an EBP project or simply want to share the review of literature you compiled, **consider publishing your findings in a professional journal** or publication. Remember journals can be in print or on-line in an electronic version. Many are fearful of the process, but it is quite easy, and there is nothing to fear. The following guide will help you through this process:

1. *First, you need an idea or topic of interest.* What types of nursing are you interested in? What field of nursing is your interest or expertise? What is your passion? What happens in your clinical work area that bothers you or peaks your curiosity so that you want to learn more about? Identify an issue. You can consult your peers, do some brainstorming, or look in the journals you receive. Many times there are sections or a page in the journal citing areas of interest in publishing, such as EBP topics, ethical issues, practice issues, and new procedures or products.
2. *Write your article* or conduct your EBP project. If you need assistance, consider a mentor. Go and speak to someone, a colleague you know who has published. Consult a previous instructor or professor.
3. *Proofread* or have others read and critique your work. Asking for insight and suggestions to improve your work may sometimes create the tone and excitement for EBP.
4. *Select a journal of interest related to your topic.* It certainly would not be appropriate to write an article or EBP proj-

ect on a pediatric issue such as immunizations and seek to publish it in a geriatric journal or an emergency/trauma journal. Select a journal that is relevant to the topic of interest.

Select a journal that is scholarly or peer reviewed. **A peer-reviewed journal is one that reviewed by a panel of experts in the field.** Peer-reviewed journals are more intensely reviewed than those reviewed by another process. This is the ideal and most respected type of publication. If this is your first submission, you may want to submit your work to a non-peer reviewed journal. Again follow the guidelines for that type of journal. There is nothing wrong with "trying the process out" with this type of journal. As you progress in your scholarly work, it is best, however, that you publish in peer-reviewed journals.

You will find the requirements for submission of a manuscript either in the journal or on the journal's Web site. To locate a journal online, just enter the name of the journal into your search engine, go to the journal's homepage, and then look for "author guidelines" or "author submissions."

Follow them exactly to avoid time delays or rejection of your submission. The journal may recommend that you submit a **"letter of query."** This is simple a letter sent to the editors telling them that you have a manuscript about a particular topic and asking if the editorial board would be interested in looking at it. If you receive a positive response, you would then submit the manuscript. If you get a negative response, you will look for another journal until you find one interested in your subject area or topic of interest.

Some examples of what you may find in the author submission guidelines are:

- The length of the manuscript.
- The type of paper and size on which it is to be submitted.
- The required font and its size.
- Spacing requirements.
- Requirements for abstracts.
- Style for bibliographies; for nursing journals, this is usually APA format.
- How to organize the body of the manuscript.
- How to handle graphics, tables, or charts.
- A description of the review process and what the timeline is for feedback to the author

These items vary by publication, and there may be a different set of guidelines for submitting your manuscript electronically. Most manuscripts are now submitted electronically. Some journals also have submission software that allows the author to establish an account and check on the status of the manuscript online at the Web site of the journal or publisher. Just remember to follow the author guidelines closely. Swanson, McCloskey, and Bodensteiner (1991) conducted a survey to determine the main reason for manuscript rejection. The highest ranked reason was that they were poorly written. This was also cited by McConnell's (2000) survey. Other reasons cited by Swanson et al. (1991) for manuscript rejection were undocumented content, unimportant content, clinically inapplicable findings, statistical problems, incorrectly interpreted data, and overly technical content technical.

Mee (2006) shares the following nine lessons on writing for publication.

1. *Be confident.* You can be a nurse author. Writing is not just for those in academic settings. Many nurses like to read about other nurses in similar situations and how they solved problems.
2. *Start small.* Don't overwhelm yourself with a large topic like pneumonia. Find an aspect of the broader topic you are passionate about, and explore it.
3. *Topic development takes time* and effort. Many nurses are intimidated and think ideas just pop into a writer's head. The truth is that many authors take a lot of time to develop their topic and focus.
4. *Gather more resources than you think you will need.* Conduct a literature search and then read all the articles you have found. Immerse yourself in the topic. Writing will be easier if you know the topic well.
5. *Know the journal you want to write for.* There are more than 150 nursing journals, both general and specialized. Choose three journals that you think your article might fit with. Then read those journals to see if the articles match your style. Follow the author guidelines and don't forget to submit a letter of interest or a query letter.
6. *Start writing in the middle.* Don't waste time trying to come up with the perfect title. Get the ideas on paper as a rough draft and then you can go back later to fix and clarify things further.
7. *Use the active rather than the passive voice.* The active voice connects with the reader. In contrast, the passive voice is

indirect, vague, and puts distance betwcen the author and the reader.

8. Multiple rewrites are the norm, so *plan for at least three rewrites.*

9. Lastly, *pay attention to detail.* Again follow the author guidelines, and put together a cleanly written and organized manuscript. Careless errors in spelling or punctuation will undermine your credibility as a writer with the editor. Then walk away and wait. Once this process is completed, and you see your name in print as an author, you will have such a sense of pride and accomplishment like you have never known. So go for it, take a chance and write (Mee, 2006).

Fast facts in a nutshell: summary

Remember that the process of publishing an article in a professional journal can be long. Sometimes, an article may not be published for at least a year. This diminishes the timeliness of important research. The best way to get current research information out to your peers in a timely fashion is to present it at a conference. That being said, whichever method you choose to share your research information, just make sure that you do. This is how the body of nursing knowledge will grow if we all share and collaborate.

REFERENCES

Center for Nursing Advocacy. (2007). What is magnet status? Accessed August 6, 2007 from http://www.nursingadvocacy.org/faq/magnet.html

Jolly, S. (2002). Raising research awareness: a strategy for nurses. *Nursing Standard, 16*(33), 33–39.

Karkos, B., & Peters, K. A. (2006). A magnet community hospital: fewer barriers to nursing research utilization. *Journal of Nursing Administration, 36*(7), 377–382.

Malloch, K. & Porter-O'Grady, T. (2006). *Introduction to evidence-based practice in nursing and health care.* Boston: Jones & Bartlett.

McConnell, E. A. (2000). Nursing publications outside the United States. *Journal of Nursing Scholarship, 32,* 87–92.

McQueen, J., Miller, C., Nivison, C., & Husband, V. (2006). An investigation into the use of a journal club for evidence-based practice.*International Journal of Therapy and Rehabilitation, 13*(7) 311–316.

Mee, C. L. (2003). Ten lessons in writing for publication. *Journal of Infusion Nursing, 26* (2), 110–113.

Melnyk, B. M. & Fineout-Overholt, E. (2005) *Evidence-based practice in nursing and health care: A guide to best practice.* Philadelphia: Lippincott, Williams & Wilkins.

Nieswiadomy, R. M. (2008). *Foundations of nursing research* (5th ed.). Upper Saddle River, NJ: Pearson.

Swanson, E. A., McCloskey, J. C., & Bodensteiner, A. (1991). Publishing opportunities for nurses: A comparison of 92 U.S. journals. *Image: Journal of Nursing Scholarship, 23,* 33–38

Wilson, S. F., & Collins, N. (2005). Video outreach journal club [electronic version]. *Rural and Remote Health,* Retrieved July 12, 2009 from http://rrh.deakin.edu.au.

Chapter 9

Example of PICO Process

Step 1: Coming up with the idea

EBP Project: The placement of post-pyloric feeding tubes in the Pediatric ICU

The interest in this topic evolved from working with the pediatric population in the Pediatric Intensive Care Unit (PICU) in examining the incidence of decreasing aspiration pneumonia in sedated ventilated patients who are being fed enterally.

Step 2: Use the PICO method: Determining the population of interest Population (P)

• Pediatric patients admitted to the Pediatric Intensive Care Unit (PICU) who are mechanically ventilated.

The Intervention (I)

• Placement of post-pyloric feeding tubes for all mechanically ventilated patients

---

Comparison (C)

- Post-pyloric feeding tubes vs. gastric feeding tubes

Outcome (O)

- Decreased incidence of aspiration pneumonia in the PICU patients on long-term mechanical ventilation

---

Step 3: Team members involved

- Maryann Godshall: project leader
- 6 nurse insertion team: Loretta Smith, Brenda Jones, Beth Sands, Jen Long, Pat Pine, and Maryann Godshall
- MD consultant: Dr. Kerrie Pinkney

Step 4: Develop a timeline

9/20/07: First meeting
9/30.07-10/30/07: Gather evidence in literature
11/1/06-5/1/07: Study period
6/1/07: Project complete

Step 5: Identify search terms

- Post-pyloric tube feedings
- Long line tube feeds
- Gastric tube feedings
- Jejunal tube feedings
- Enteral tube feedings

- Aspiration pneumonia
- Transpyloric tube feedings

Step 6: Determine search engines

- CINAHL
- EBSCO
- Ovid on-line
- Cochrane data base
- PubMed

**Step 7: Gather the evidence and prepare an
          evidence table**

Below is an example of just 2 research articles found for this project

TABLE 9.1   Example of an Evidence Table

Reference	Purpose/ Hypothesis Research Question	Sample	Classification of evidence	Method	Results
Mcquire, W., & McEwan, P. (2006). Transpyloric versus gastric tube feeding for preterm infants. The Cochrane Library. Ovid on-line	Does feeding via the transpyloric route *vs.* the gastric route improve feeding tolerance, and growth and development without increasing adverse consequences?	8 studies undertaken from 1970s through early 1980s. Very low birth weight infants (less than 1500 grams). Only infants grown appropriately for gestational age were used. Some of the infants on respiratory or ventilatory support were not included	3A- systematic review of homogeneity of case-control studies	Randomized or quasirandomized controlled trials comparing transpyloric *vs.* gastric tube feedings in preterm infants	No evidence of benefit of transpyloric feeding in preterm infants. There were adverse effects found and therefore feeding preterm infants via the transpyloric route *cannot* be recommended.

Joffe, A.R., Grant, M. Wondg, B., & Gresiuk, C. (2000). Validation of blind transpyloric feeding tube placement techniques in pediatric intensive care, Pediatric Critical Care Medicine, 1(2), 151-155.	Blind Insertion of transpyloric feeding tubes in pediatric intensive care is highly successful	Children in pediatric intensive care without fudoplication, pharyngeal trauma, or gastric ulceration whose intensivists requested TP feedings. Patients who were hemodynamically unstable to tolerate the procedure and those who had an absent cough while not endotracheally intubated were also excluded. Patients were <17 yrs old. Average age 0.73-198 months of age	2C- Outcomes Research	Prospective Interventional Study	71 feedings tubes inserted in 38 patients over a 9-month period from 2/99-10/99. Success rate of blind transpyloric feeding tube insertion was 88.7%. The average insertion time took an average of 5 minutes.

(continued)

Reference	Purpose/ Hypothesis Research Question	Sample	Classification of evidence	Method	Results
		and weighed 3-70 kg. The diagnosis included post-op heart surgery (n=15), resp failure (n=7), septic shock (n=4), coma (n=4), traumatic brain injury (n=3), airway maintenance (n=3), and burns (n=2). 69% were ventilated, 15.5% had pharmacologic paralysis, 78.9% has continuous infusion of sedation. Tubes were nasally placed in 94.4% and orally placed in 5.6% of patients.			

Step 8: Summarize your evidence

- The evidence shows that transpyloric feeding tubes can be easily placed by the blind method easily (<5 minutes) and successfully (88.7%) in the PICU.
- This method should NOT be used in the Neonatal Intensive Care Unit (NICU).

Step 9: Practice Implications

- The placement of transpyloric tube feedings can be placed easily and successfully in the PICU.
- Evidence shows that transpyloric tube feedings decreases the incidence of aspiration pneumonia.
- To decrease the incidence of aspiration pneumonia in the PICU, the placement of transpyloric tube feedings should be implemented.

Author Comment: This is just one example of an evidence based practice project done. You can tailor the process to meet your institutions needs. Not all instutions rate the evidence. If you do rate the evidence, there are numerous rating scales available for you to use.

Glossary

Abstract   A brief summary about the research article. It should contain the purpose, methods, and major findings of the study. By reading an abstract, the researcher should be able to understand the basic highlights of a research article

Aesthetic knowledge   Abstract information that gives us an appreciation of the deeper meaning of the situation. In takes an inductive approach to knowledge acquisition.

Assumptions   Statements and principles that are taken as truth, based on a person's values and beliefs.

Bias   Occurs when researchers interject their personal beliefs into the study. This is a deviation from the true results of the study.

Biophysiologic measure   A measure that includes both in vivo and in vitro measures. A biophysiologic method is one that tests an instrument of some kind.

Bivariate study   A study with two variables. One variable is usually the dependent variable, and one is the independent variable.

Blinding   Occurs during the research process when the subjects do not know if they are in the experimental group or the control group.

Borrowed theories   Theories taken from another discipline, for example psychology, and applied to nursing questions and research problems.

Bracketing   The process by which researchers identify their own personal biases about the phenomenon of interest to clarify their personal experiences and beliefs that may alter or reflect what is heard and reported.

Case studies   In-depth examinations of people or groups of people. In a case study, institutions or facilities could be examined, for example an in-patient psychiatric unit.

Clinical practice guidelines   Systematic reviews that put a large amount of evidence into a manageable and usable format. They give specific practice recommendations for making EBP decisions, address the issues relevant to a clinical decision, which include balancing the benefit and risks of a EBP decision, and are developed to help guide clinical practice even when there is limited available evidence.

Community based-participatory action research   A method of research which involves the community to take an active part in the research process. The community takes an active part in all stages of the research process, including planning, conducting, implementing, and evaluating.

Comparative studies   Studies that look at the difference between intact groups on some dependent variable of interest.

Comparison   This occurs when an individual assesses the similar and dissimilar characteristics of a particular object, situation, or research variable.

Concepts   The building blocks of theories that are used to describe phenomenon or a group of phenomena. A concept gives some degree of classification or categorization.

Conceptual model   In research, similar to a conceptual framework. It is a set of abstract and general concepts that are assembled to address a phenomenon of central interest.

Confidence intervals   Reflect the degree of risk researchers are willing to take of being wrong. With a 95% confidence interval, the researcher accepts the probability that they will be wrong only 5 times out of 100.

Constructs Higher level concepts that are derived from theories and that represent nonobservable behaviors.

Control or comparison group The group not receiving the intervention of interest or the group with which the experimental group is compared.

Correlational studies The researcher examines the strength of the relationship between variables by determining how the change in one variable is associated with the changes in another variable.

Cross-sectional A survey or study that looks at people at one point in time.

Cumulative Index to Nursing and Allied Health Literature (CINAHL) First published in 1961, and still published today, it covers nursing and allied health journals, including dental hygiene, nutrition, occupational therapy, physical therapy, physician's assistant, and respiratory therapy journals. It is an index to written and online articles.

Database A collection of data or information stored in a computer. You can think of it as a electronic filing system.

Dependent variable The "effect" or that which is influenced by the independent variable. The dependent variable can also be called the criterion, or outcome variable.

Descriptive studies Describe things or objects. They describe the phenomena of interest or the relationship between variables. This is different from an exploratory study in that there would be information in the literature about the phenomena of interest in a descriptive study.

Descriptive theory Empirically driven theory that "describes or classifies specific dimensions or characteristics of individuals, groups, situations, or events by summarizing commonalities found in discrete observations."

Directional hypothesis Shows that there is an expected direction in the relationship between variables.

Double blinding A two-way process in which neither the researcher nor the subject knows who received the intervention and who is in the control group in a study.

Effect size   The magnitude of the impact of an intervention or variable is expected to have on the outcome.

Emic   Intrinsic or from the internal perspective of a culture.

Empirical knowledge   What we know through our physical senses; something we can hear, touch, taste, and see. This is best handled through quantitative methods of knowledge discovery.

Ethical knowledge   That by which we make moment-to-moment decisions. What is right, what should be done, and what is good. This directs our personal conduct in life.

Ethnography   A qualitative study that explores the cultural aspects of a particular group of informants.

Ethnonursing   A qualitative study that explores the cultural aspects of a particular group of informants in relation to nursing or how they perceive aspects of nursing care.

Etic   Extrinsic, or from the external perspective of a culture.

Experimental group   The group of subjects receiving the intervention of interest.

Explanatory research studies   The researcher searches for causal explanations. This method is much more rigorous than exploratory or descriptive research. The researcher provides an explanation for the relationships that are found among the phenomena.

Explode   A technique used if you want to expand your database search to include other terms. This is done by including additional narrower subject headings to your key word list.

Exploratory studies   Conducted when little is known about the phenomena.

Extraneous variables   Variables that are not under investigation or examination, but may or may not be relevant to or interfere with the study. Extraneous variables may be controlled or uncontrolled by the researcher. The researcher should identify any extraneous variables when possible to avoid interference with the study or cause any adverse or unplanned effect. Extraneous variables may also be called confounding variables, intervening variables, or mediating variables.

Feminist research Research that focuses on gender domination and discrimination within patriarchal societies. These researchers seek to establish a nonexploitive relationship with their informants and to conduct research that transforms these perceived boundaries.

Field notes Notes the researcher may take about an interview to help to remember later remember facts that were important to the study (usually done after the interview is completed).

Focus Used to narrow your search using certain computer databases.

Grand theories Complex and broad in scope. They try to explain broad areas and include many concepts that are not usually grounded in empirical data (data gathered through the senses using objective measurement) or evidence.

Grounded theory Research studies in which data is collected and analyzed. After that, a theory is developed that is grounded in the data.

Hawthorne effect The subjects in a study change their behavior, actions, or answers to questions when they know they are being studied. They may answer a question the "way they think" the researcher wants it answered as opposed to how they really feel.

Health Insurance Portability and Accountability Act of 1996 (HIPPA) A law passed by the United States Congress that created national standards for electronic medical information to keep health information private. An institution. such as a hospital, can disclose individually identifiable health information (IIHI) from its records if a patient signs an authorization gaining access.

Hyperlink Occurs when one clicks on the Web address or words given in a text that will automatically connect your computer (link) with the article of interest. These can be used to make access to online information easier.

Hypothesis   In research, a prediction about the relationship between two or more variables.

Immersion   A research technique in which the researcher spends time at the place of interest, so that the participants or informants gain trust in the researcher or simply get to know the researcher and hopefully be more open in discussions.

Independent variable   The "cause," or the variable that influences the dependent variable.

Index Medicus   This publication ceased in December 2004 with Volume 45. This index is the best known index of medical literature. The first volume was published in 1879. It is still available on library shelves. In 1997 this data base became available for free on the Internet through MEDLINE.

Instrumental case study   Used when a researcher is pursuing insight into an issue or wants to challenge some generalization and the particular case was instrumental or of utmost importance to the subject being studied.

Integrative review   Generalizations about substantive issues from a set of studies that have direct bearing on those issues. Integrative reviews are scholarly papers that synthesize published studies and articles to answer questions about phenomena of interest. They are frequently found in peer-reviewed professional publications.

Interrater reliability   A term used when you have two or more individuals or "coders" gathering information during a study. It is the degree to which they agree. For judging purposes, it is a consensus, or how often they agree on a given score. In research, it is how often two observers agree on a given item and the level of agreement between them.

Intervention   What you want to do with the defined patient population. A nursing intervention is a nursing measure that you physically do to your patient.

In vitro   A measure taken from a participant in a study and then subjected to laboratory analysis, such as the measuring of a potassium level, bacterial count, or a tissue biopsy.

In vivo   A measure that is performed directly within or on a living being. (Examples include blood pressure, heart rate, or respiratory rate).

Key informant   A person who is knowledgeable about the population of interest. He or she might also be able to provide the researcher with access to the designated population.

Key words   Terms that describe the subject of interest.

Landmark studies   Studies that may be older than five years but are paramount to the direction of study of the topic. These studies are significant to the understanding of the topic.

Letter of query   A letter of query is simple a letter sent to the members of the editorial board of a publication asking if they would be interested in looking at your specific article.

Level of significance   Measures how much evidence we have against the null hypothesis. It is written as a "p-value." If the p-value is less than 0.05, the result is significant. If the p value is greater than 0.05, the result is not considered significant.

Longitudinal survey or study   A study that follows subjects over a period of time.

Metaanalysis   The process of combining results of studies into a measureable format, statistically estimating the effects of proposed interventions, and critically reviewing them to minimize bias.

Metaparadigm   A primary phenomenon of interest to a particular discipline. The nursing metaparadigm usually consists of four components: the person, the environment, health, and how the concept of nursing fits into the metaparadigm.

Methodological studies   The researchers look at "the method." This is use mainly to test instruments or look at the development, testing, and evaluation of research instruments.

Middle-range theories   Theories that focus on only a piece of reality or human experience, involving a selected number of concepts, such as theories of stress.

Narrative research   A type of research that allows people to "tell their own stories" to uncover their motivations, desires, or feelings in a multitude of settings.

Nondirectional hypothesis   Shows no direction between variables.

Null hypothesis   The complete lack of or absence of a relationship between the variables.

Nursing Studies Indexes (NSI)   This index provides an annotate guide to English-language reports of studies and historical and bibliographical materials about nursing. It is helpful when looking for material published during the first half of the twentieth century (1900-1959).

Outcome   The end result. What one wants to accomplish or measure.

Peer-reviewed journal   A publication in which all articles are reviewed by experts in the field of the research topic. The article must pass the test of usually more than one expert or reviewer before it is accepted for publication. The review process usually takes place in a blinded fashion, in which reviewers do not know the author. All identifying author criteria and credentials are omitted from the article prior to the review process.

Personal knowledge   Concerns the inner experience we have. It is the shared human experience and humanistic qualities of knowing.

Phenomenology   A method that explores the meaning of human experience through the "lived experience" of the individual.

Pilot study   A small-scale trial run of a larger research study usually using a smaller number of subjects.

Population   The group of individuals you want to examine. It can be infants, toddlers, preschoolers, adolescents, or adults of a particular age. It can also be a group of individuals, such as psychiatric patients with the diagnosis of schizophrenia.

Practice theories   More specific than middle-range theories, they produce specific directions or guidelines for practice. An example of a practice theory is the Theories of End-of-Life Decision Making

Prescriptive theories   Theories that address nursing therapeutics and the outcomes of interventions. A prescriptive theory includes propositions that call for change and predict the consequences of a certain strategy for nursing intervention.

Primary data sources   Would be eyewitness accounts of the time being studied. Studies by people who were actually present or the person who conducted the research or wrote about it.

Problem statement   Formally addresses the problem being examined. It is the "what" of the study. It should include the scope of the research problem, the specific population being studied, the independent and dependent variables, and the goal or question the study is trying to answer. It can be in the form of a declarative statement or an interrogatory question.

Purpose   The reason the problem is being examined. It is the "why" of the study.

Purposive sampling   A sampling method in which researchers use their own judgment in selecting people who will be representative of the group that the researcher is interested in exploring. For example, the researcher may go to a battered woman's shelter to study the lived experience of abusive relationships.

Qualitative research   Research that is considered subjective and is more flexible in design. It describes an individual experience. It usually has a written narrative or verbal description. There usually are fewer participants in the study sample.

Quantitative research   A type of research that is considered more objective. It imposes tight control over the research situation and is often a more rigorous and controlled design. It generalizes findings and frequently includes numbers, facts, and figures. When you think of quantitative research; think quantity. The sample study usually has a large number of participants or subjects.

Quasi-experimental design   Fulfills the same rules for an experimental design except that there is no comparison group.

Randomization   A procedure that assures that every subject has an equal chance of being chosen for the experiment.

Reliability   The ability to measure what you want to measure on subsequent experiences.

Research problem   An area of concern or one in which there may be a gap in knowledge or literature that is in need of a solution.

Research questions   Statements of the specific query or investigation to answer or address a research problem. In some cases, they are a direct rewording of the statement of purpose, which is then phrased as a question.

Research utilization   Applying a single research study or part of a study to something unrelated to the original research.

Retrospective study   A study that looks backward in time to data already obtained and on record. This type of study can be done by reviewing charts of previously collected data.

Saturation   When common themes are found in qualitative research and no new information is obtained. This is called the point of saturation.

Search engine   A search engine is an information retrieval system that is stored on a computer system such as the World Wide Web. One of the most popular today is Google™.

Secondary sources   A view or account of an event by someone other than an eye-witness.

Scope   Clicking on the scope icon ℹ enables you to check the scope of a term and its synonyms.

Single blinding   A one-way process in which subjects do not know if they are in the experimental group or the control group.

Standard deviation   Shows the average amount of deviation of values away from the mean. A standard deviation is a useful variability index for describing a distribution and interpreting individual scores in relation to other scores in the sample.

Systematic review   A state-of-the-art summary of all the research information available at a given time on a particular subject. This is not a literature review, but a review of actual research studies. Items in a systematic review all address a specific clinical question.

Truncation   Used to find words with a similar stem. A common symbol or truncations is the (*). This is used to find variant word endings.

Univariate study   A study with just one variable.

Validity   The ability to measure what it is supposed to or intended to measure.

Vulnerable subjects   Special groups of people in a research study whose rights need to be protected because they are unable or incapable of providing an informed consent. For example, children, unconscious adults, mentally retarded or emotionally disabled people, severely ill or physically disabled people, or people who are terminally ill. Pregnant women are included because possible unintended side effects to the unborn child, who is considered vulnerable.

Index

217